General Surgery Boards
Case-Based Review

Scarlett Hao • Alex Dai
Michael Honaker

General Surgery
Boards Case-Based
Review

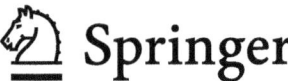 Springer

Scarlett Hao
Surgery
East Carolina University
Greenville, NC, USA

Alex Dai
Surgery
East Carolina University
Greenville, NC, USA

Michael Honaker
Surgery
East Carolina University
Greenville, NC, USA

ISBN 978-3-031-85630-3   ISBN 978-3-031-85631-0   (eBook)
https://doi.org/10.1007/978-3-031-85631-0

This Springer imprint is published by the registered company Springer Nature
Switzerland AG
The registered company address is: Gewerbestrasse 11, 6330 Cham, Switzerland

If disposing of this product, please recycle the paper.

To all of the patients who are the best teachers of surgical trainees, and to all of the mentors who support the next generation of surgeon physicians.

Acknowledgments

We would like to thank the general surgery residents and faculty of the East Carolina University program for their participation in the curriculum from which the structure of this book is derived. The authors have no conflicts of interest to declare that are relevant to the content of this book.

About the Book

Like most surgical textbooks, the content of this book are divided into the subspecialties of the field. However, this categorization is based primarily on the presenting pathology of each case. The sequelae of each case may dive into crossover sections just as real cases and real exam setting scenarios may go. The answers to each question are written in active voice to help the reader practice verbalizing as if performing in an oral boards setting. Repetitive steps such as seeking multidisciplinary conference for all cancer cases or performing the ABC evaluation for trauma patients are repeated to help internalize what may be secondhand in clinical practice but easy to forget to verbalize in a test scenario. Where possible, multiple options for correct answers are presented, especially in controversial arenas. Otherwise, the answers are dictated by the available literature and guidelines which are provided in the Additional Reading section following each chapter. This book does not include diagnostic challenges such as reading radiographs or interpreting a lab panel, as the focus is on decision-making given a particular situation. The decision to pursue a line of work-up in order to make a diagnosis is sometimes included if felt to be frequently tested. Along this guiding principle, relevant bloodwork values and conclusive radiographic findings are directly provided. The reader is encouraged to submit feedback to help develop future editions as the practice of medicine and surgery evolves.

Contents

Abbreviations

IV	intravenous line
TXA	tranexamic acid
FAST	focused assessment with sonography in trauma
REBOA	resuscitative endovascular balloon occlusion of the aorta
IVC	inferior vena cava
SMA	superior mesenteric artery
ICU	intensive care unit
CO_2	carbon dioxide
FiO_2	fraction of inspired oxygen
CXR	chest x-ray
ARDS	acute respiratory distress syndrome
EKG	electrocardiogram
SVT	supraventricular tachycardia
ROSC	return of spontaneous circulation
GI	gastrointestinal
TBSA	total body surface area
CT	computed tomography
CEA	carcinoembryonic antigen
Ca 19-9	cancer antigen 19-9
AFP	alpha-fetoprotein
HCC	hepatocellular carcinoma
UNOS	United Network for Organ Sharing
GIST	gastrointestinal stromal tumor
NSAID	non-steroidal anti-inflammatory drug
CRP	c-reactive protein

BMI	body mass index
TIPS	transjugular intrahepatic portosystemic shunt
MSLT-2	Multicenter Selective Lymphadenectomy Trial II
BI-RADS	Breast Imaging Reporting & Data System
ACOSOG Z-11	American College of Surgeons Oncology Group Z0011
BRCA	breast cancer gene
AVF	arteriovenous fistula
ABI	ankle-brachial indices
PTH	parathyroid hormone
PTHRP	parathyroid hormone related protein
beta-hCG	beta-human chorionic gonadotropin

List of Figures

List of Tables

Trauma and Critical Care

1

Case Scenario

You are the trauma team leader receiving a 24-year-old woman who was the restrained passenger in a motor vehicle collision traveling at highway speeds. She was hypotensive en route but responsive to crystalloid.

What's Your Next Step?

Prior to patient arrival, you put on personal protective equipment; brief the trauma team; ensure ancillary staff are prepared including radiology, laboratory, respiratory, and the operating room personnel, as well as consultant specialists; and delegate roles. After the patient arrives and is transferred to the bed, you receive handoff from the transport team and begin with your airway, breathing, circulation assessment, ensuring the patient has a protected airway, bilateral and adequate ventilation, and two large bore intravenous (IV) lines in addition to an updated vitals check.

The patient does respond verbally and appropriately but is in distress, has clear breath sounds bilaterally, and has the following vital signs: heart rate of 130, blood pressure of 80/50 mmHg, and O2 saturation of 96% on nasal cannula. The transport team tells you that the patient is healthy with no comorbidities, allergies, or

S. Hao et al., *General Surgery Boards Case-Based Review*, https://doi.org/10.1007/978-3-031-85631-0_1

medications, and that they have already administered tranexamic acid (TXA) and two liters of normal saline.

You transfuse two units of uncrossed blood and complete your primary survey, assessing for obvious injuries that may explain why she is in shock while also protecting the spine and ensuring the patient is kept warm. You send off stat bloodwork. You also obtain updated vitals.

The patient's tachycardia and hypotension improve after transfusion but do not normalize. You see no obvious injuries.

What's the Working Diagnosis?

You are concerned about an internal source of hemorrhage. You perform a bedside focused assessment with sonography in trauma (FAST) exam, which is positive in all three abdominal views. As you complete your FAST exam, the patient's blood pressure drops again. You order additional blood to be transfused and consent the patient for urgent exploratory laparotomy.

Operative Steps

Trauma Laparotomy Principles

1. Position the patient supine with arms abducted; decompress the stomach and bladder; prep from chin to thigh; consider having autotransfusion equipment available if possible.
2. Begin with midline celiotomy from xiphoid to pubis, eviscerate the small bowel, and immediately pack all four quadrants.
3. Remove packs quadrant by quadrant and control bleeding (Table 1.1).
4. Address injuries as they are found but explore the abdominal cavity systematically (Table 1.2).
5. Communicate with anesthesia and evaluate patient stability and injury pattern for definitive intervention and closure versus temporary abdominal closure (Table 1.3).

Table 1.1 Options for vascular control of major aortic or caval injuries

Aortic control	Cross-clamp descending thoracic aorta through left anterolateral thoracotomy
	Insertion of resuscitative endovascular balloon occlusion of the aorta (REBOA) catheter with deployment supraceliac, suprarenal, or infrarenal
	Open lesser omentum with stomach and distal esophagus retracted to the left and apply manual pressure or use an aortic compressor or a clamp at the aortic hiatus
	Perform a left medial visceral rotation to access the supramesocolic aorta
	Elevate the transverse mesocolon and open a mesenteric window to access the inframesocolic or infrarenal aorta
	Incise the peritoneum to expose the bifurcation of the infrarenal aorta
	Perform a femoral cutdown below the inguinal ligament to access femoral artery
IVC control	Perform median sternotomy to access the intrapericardial inferior vena cava (IVC)
	Divide triangular, falciform, and gastrohepatic ligaments to mobilize the liver to access the suprahepatic IVC
	Perform a right medial visceral rotation to access the infrahepatic IVC
	Incise the peritoneum at the pelvic inlet to control the common iliac vessels
	Perform Pringle maneuver to control portal vein

Table 1.2 Systematic exploration of the abdominal cavity

Solid organs	Palpate over the dome of the liver and the undersurface as well
	Enter the lesser sac to evaluate the pancreas body
	Visualize any blood welling from the left upper quadrant or palpate the spleen
Hollow organs	Elevate the transverse mesocolon and identify the ligament of Treitz
	Run the small bowel to the cecum
	Inspect the large bowel from cecum to upper rectum at the peritoneal reflection
	Further inspection of the large bowel may require right or left medial visceral rotation by releasing the white line of Toldt
	Examine anterior stomach as well as the posterior stomach by entering the lesser sac
	Perform Kocher maneuver to evaluate the duodenum

(continued)

Table 1.2   (continued)

Retroperitoneum	Eviscerate the bowel and perform bilateral medial visceral rotation as needed to inspect bilateral zone 2 retroperitoneum for presence of hematoma and any change in its size or appearance
	Elevate the transverse mesocolon and inspect the root of the mesentery to evaluate for a zone 1 hematoma
	Retract intestines to the epigastrium and visually inspect the pelvis and sacral promontory for a zone 3 hematoma
	Inspect bilateral hemidiaphragms

Table 1.3   Indications for damage control approach in trauma laparotomy

Hemodynamic instability
Pelvic fractures with expanding pelvic bleeding
Extra-abdominal injuries requiring intervention
Multiple high severity injuries in multiple categories (i.e., vascular, hollow organ, solid organ, retroperitoneal)
Inability to close without undue tension

Operative Pearl

Hemorrhage control outweighs enteric control.

On exploration, you encounter a constellation of injuries:

Operative Steps

Retroperitoneal Hematoma

1. Explore all zone 1 hematomas and all penetrating hematomas regardless of zone, but explore only expanding blunt trauma zone 2 and three hematomas.
2. Obtain proximal and distal control (Table 1.1).
3. Rule out aortic and major arterial source first.
4. Rule out major venous source second.
5. Repair vascular injuries primarily with running 4–0 nonabsorbable monofilament sutures in transverse direction, or with patch or graft.

6. Temporize with shunt if patient is too unstable or injury too complex for repair but ligation is not an option.

Operative Pearl

Having collaterals allows safe ligation: i.e., the origin of the celiac may be ligated but not the superior mesenteric artery (SMA).

Hepatic Injury

1. Evaluate location and degree of hepatic injury.
2. Obtain vascular control.
3. Repair lacerations with 2–0 chromic suture or ligate transected biliary radicals and blood vessels or pack and suture omental flaps into deep lacerations.
4. Resect destructive injury not amenable to repair.
5. Widely drain.

Splenic Injury (Splenectomy)

1. Enter the lesser sac through the gastrocolic ligament and divide this ligament to reach the spleen.
2. Medialize the spleen by freeing the splenocolic, gastrosplenic, splenorenal, and splenophrenic ligaments (Fig. 1.1).
3. Isolate and transect the hilum with a vascular staple load (alternatively, suture ligate each vessel).
4. Leave a closed suction drain near the pancreatic tail.

Duodenal Injury

1. Evaluate full length of the duodenum after Kocher maneuver from pylorus to the ligament of Treitz.
2. For a hematoma, opt for conservative management if less than 50% of the lumen is compromised.

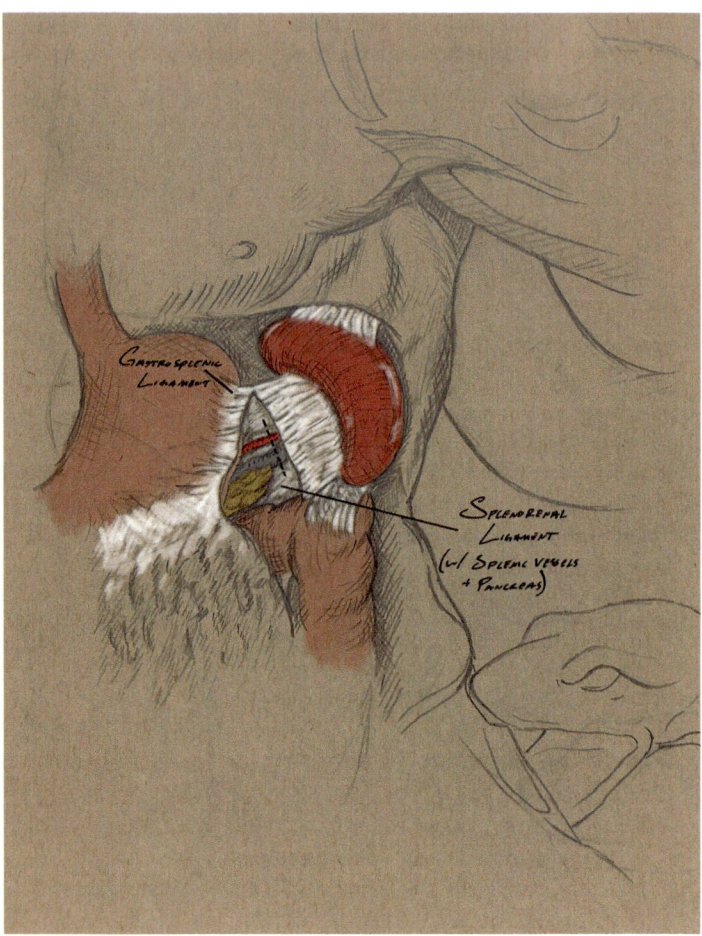

Fig. 1.1 Splenic ligaments and hilum

- Incise and drain a hematoma if there is significant luminal obstruction without mucosal violation and close the incision.
3. For a laceration, debride back to healthy tissue edges, evaluate ampulla involvement, and opt for simple transverse repair if less than 50% of the circumference has been violated.

- For a larger laceration not amenable to simple repair, perform either duodenojejunostomy or duodenal exclusion with distal reconstruction (gastrojejunostomy or more distal duodenojejunostomy).
4. For injury involving the ampulla, temporize with wide drainage including biliary drainage and consider intraoperative consultation of hepatobiliary expertise or transfer to a center with such expertise.
5. Consider feeding access as well as decompression and drainage tubes.

Small Intestine Injury

1. Suture repair serosal injuries and full thickness lacerations involving less than 50% of the circumference.
2. Resect segments with significant damage to either the bowel or its associated mesentery.
3. Delay anastomosis if opting for damage control management.

Operative Pearl

When suturing the gastrointestinal tract, full thickness closure should be done in two layers.

Large Intestine Injury

1. Suture repair serosal injuries and full thickness lacerations involving less than 50% of the circumference.
2. Resect segments with significant damage to either the bowel or its associated mesentery.
3. Delay anastomosis if opting for damage control.
4. Consider diversion if opting for anastomosis or performing end colostomy and mucous fistula for long stumps.

Sequela

You successfully control hemorrhage and resect injured intestine, but due to hemodynamic instability, you place a temporary abdominal closure and take the patient to the intensive care unit (ICU) for resuscitation. You stabilize the patient and return for a second look in 48 h with definitive intervention and closure.

On second look, you are able to carefully examine all organs and identify additional injuries:

Operative Steps

Gastric Injury

1. Evaluate anterior and posterior stomach by dividing the gastrocolic ligament in order to enter the lesser sac, taking care to protect the short gastric and epiploic blood supply.
2. Debride wound edges of any lacerations back to healthy mucosa.
3. Repair using absorbable suture in interrupted seromuscular bites.
4. Perform pyloroplasty if the laceration involves the pylorus (see Chap. 3).
5. Resect destructive injury not amenable to repair, such as those which have left portions of the stomach devascularized which require partial or total gastrectomy with reconstruction.
6. Consider feeding access as well as decompression and drainage tubes.

Pancreatic Injury

1. Enter the lesser sac if a hematoma overlying the pancreas is visualized.
2. Evaluate for parenchymal and duct injury.
3. If the duct is not injured, leave drains.

4. If the duct is injured, assess if the injury is lateral or medial to the SMA.
5. If lateral to the SMA, perform distal pancreatectomy with or without splenectomy (see Chap. 10) and widely drain.
6. If medial to the SMA, temporize with wide drainage and consider intraoperative consultation of hepatobiliary expertise or transfer to a center with such expertise.

Operative Pearl

Intraoperative ultrasound can help identify underlying ductal injury.

Rectal Injury

1. Identify intraperitoneal rectal injury during exploratory laparotomy and extraperitoneal rectal injury via proctoscopy with the patient in lithotomy or frog-legged position.
2. Manage intraperitoneal rectal injury akin to colonic injuries.
3. Manage extraperitoneal rectal injury with diversion (perform transanal repairs only if accessible and with appropriate expertise).

Bladder Injury

1. Repair intraperitoneal dome injuries not involving the trigone in two layers with absorbable suture and leave a pelvic drain.
2. Consult urology for assistance with injury proximate to the ureters.

Renal Injury

1. Obtain vascular control of the hilum.
2. Repair capsular tears with absorbable suture.
3. Consider nephrectomy in unsalvageable severe injuries.

Diaphragm Injury

1. Reduce and evaluate any herniated contents through the diaphragmatic defect.
2. Close the defect with nonabsorbable suture with a chest tube in place.

> **Operative Pearl**
>
> Be familiar with nonoperative management of injuries identified clinically or radiographically.

Case Scenario

Your next trauma patient is a 28-year-old male football player who arrives after sustaining a gunshot wound to the neck. The only known medical history is that he has been told he has a large heart. He has two large bore IVs and is already receiving one liter crystalloid bolus. He is sitting upright, drooling, and reports pain with swallowing. There is a blood-soaked pressure dressing at his left anterior neck. He is saturating 80% on 10 L nasal cannula and is breathing at a shallow and rapid rate. His blood pressure is 95/55 mmHg. He has no other injuries noted on exposure.

What's the Working Diagnosis?

You are concerned about potential injury to the trachea and esophagus, in addition to possible vascular injury. You are also worried about imminent airway compromise and airway failure.

What's Your Next Step?

You prioritize securing the airway, with consideration for awake intubation or awake tracheostomy.

However, the patient acutely decompensates with declining mentation and dropping oxygen saturation. Your airway team is unable to intubate successfully despite all adjuncts including gum bougie, video laryngoscopy, etc. You decide to perform emergent cricothyroidotomy.

Operative Steps

Cricothyroidotomy

1. Using palpated landmarks, incise and dissect down to the cricothyroid membrane.
2. Incise the membrane and pass a size 6 or smaller endotracheal tube into the trachea.
3. Inflate the balloon and confirm end-tidal carbon dioxide (CO_2) and chest expansion.

Sequela

You secure the airway successfully. The patient's oxygen saturation improves. The blood pressure transiently improves with transfusion but the neck wound continues to bleed. The wound is located on the left neck just anterior to the sternocleidomastoid muscle below the angle of the jaw and above the cricoid cartilage. You obtain plain films which reveal a retained missile in the central neck without cervical spinal injury. You ensure ongoing resuscitation, intravenous access, and invasive monitoring, and plan to take the patient for urgent neck exploration as well as formalization of the cricothyroidotomy to a tracheostomy.

Operative Steps

Neck Exploration

1. Position the patient supine with arms tucked and neck extended (except in spinal injury) and head turned away from the injury site.
2. Make longitudinal incision along the sternocleidomastoid muscle from the sternum to mastoid.
3. Divide strap muscles to expose the carotid sheath, the esophagus, and the trachea for evaluation for injury.

Tracheostomy

1. Incise 2 fingerbreadths above the sternal notch.
2. Divide the median raphe.
3. Divide or retract the thyroid isthmus.
4. Confirm operative steps to reduce fire risk: disconnect electro-cautery, have water available, reduce fraction of inspired oxygen (FiO_2).
5. Deflate the endotracheal tube balloon, retract the endotracheal tube, and incise the trachea at the second ring.
6. Insert the tracheostomy and confirm end-tidal CO_2 prior to securement and remove the endotracheal tube.

Sequela

You retrieve the retained missile and identify a small laceration to the common carotid which is easily repaired. The esophagus and trachea are otherwise uninjured. You successfully convert the cricothyroidotomy to a tracheostomy.

You admit the patient to the ICU. The patient continues to have a high FiO_2 requirement and a chest X-ray (CXR) reveals right lower lobe infiltrates. On repeat bloodwork, the patient continues to have a leukocytosis. The patient spikes a fever.

What's the Working Diagnosis?

Although pulmonary infiltrates after blunt trauma may be contusions, this would not be consistent with this patient's mechanism of trauma. You are concerned about pneumonia or aspiration pneumonitis or mucus plugging. Acute respiratory distress syndrome (ARDS) is less likely given the unilaterality.

What's the Treatment Plan?

You opt to perform a bedside bronchoscopy with bronchoalveolar lavage and obtain consent.

Operative Steps

Bronchoscopy

1. Ensure staff and equipment are at bedside and that the patient is continuously monitored.
2. Maximize FiO2 and adjust ventilator settings.
3. Administer topical lidocaine and IV sedatives.
4. Insert the bronchoscope through the tracheostomy.
5. Inspect for airway appearance and any secretions as you travel to the target area.
6. Instill 20–50 cc of saline and suction with a suction trap in place, and repeat this three to five times, withdrawing at least 30% of the instilled volume.
7. Send the specimen for culture.

Sequela

The patient is adequately treated for aspiration pneumonitis and weans off the ventilator. Invasive lines are discontinued.

The bedside nurse pages you abruptly to tell you that the patient is extremely tachycardic after getting up to work with therapy. His heart rate is 168 bpm and his cuff pressure is 83/55 mmHg. You appropriately order an electrocardiogram (EKG) which reveals narrow complex tachycardia.

What's the Working Diagnosis?

You are concerned about an unstable supraventricular tachycardia (SVT). You plan for synchronized cardioversion. You ensure pads are applied and the defibrillator is set to synchronize. You administer a sedative and a 50 joule shock.

The patient's SVT normalizes briefly and then decompensates into an irregular wide complex tachycardia with no discernible pattern. The bedside nurse reports no pulse.

You are concerned that the rhythm is now ventricular fibrillation.

What's the Next Step?

You call a hospital code and immediately begin cardiopulmonary resuscitation. You attempt to shock the patient with 150 joules and then continue chest compressions.

What's the Working Diagnosis?

Hypovolemia, hemorrhage, hyper−/hypokalemia, hypoxia, thrombosis, tamponade, pneumothorax, and toxins are all on the differential. You successfully achieve return of spontaneous circulation (ROSC). Further evaluation by cardiology indicates the patient likely has hypertrophic cardiomyopathy.

It is three weeks later and the patient has since been able to wean off the vent and is recuperating in the rehabilitation unit. You are paged to see the patient due to a report that blood was noted from the trachea.

What's the Working Diagnosis?

You are concerned about the most dangerous possibility, which is a tracheo-innominate fistula, but it may also be an upper gastrointestinal (GI) bleed, any oropharyngeal source of blood which may be aspirated, or a parenchymal source of hemoptysis.

You present promptly to assess the patient and the patient acutely coughs up a large volume of bright red blood from the trachea. The hemorrhage does not appear to cease. The patient's heart rate is 125 and blood pressure is 80/50 mmHg.

What's the Next Step?

You intubate the patient from above and remove the cuffless trach and apply the Utley maneuver. You quickly take the patient to the operating room, activating massive transfusion protocol along the way. You ensure there are two large bore IVs and that transfusion or crystalloid administration is started.

What's the Treatment Plan?

The patient needs ligation and division of the innominate artery and repair of the trachea with a flap. If vascular expertise is available, stenting across the fistula may be an option.

Case Scenario

The ambulance brings to your trauma bay a 16-year-old male who was rescued from a burning home. On your primary survey, you note that the patient does respond verbally and appropriately but sounds hoarse and coughs up carbonaceous sputum. He has breath sounds bilaterally and has the following vital signs: heart rate of 115, blood pressure of 120/60 mmHg, respiratory rate of 20, and O2 saturation of 96% on nasal cannula. The transport team tells you that the patient is healthy with no comorbidities, allergies, or medications and weighs 70 kg. Two peripheral large bore IVs are already in place. A quick survey reveals severely burned skin on the patient's upper arms and chest and upper back.

What's Your Working Diagnosis?

You are concerned about airway burn injury in addition to the potential for carbon monoxide poisoning and other thermal burn injuries. You estimate 36–40% total body surface area (TBSA) burned.

What's the Next Step?

You initiate weight-based fluid resuscitation (Table 1.4) and plan for awake laryngoscopy, looking for signs such as edema, debris, ulcers, or mucosal slough.

You do note significant edema and blistering in the airway. You plan on intubation.

Table 1.4 Formulas for calculating fluid requirements in patients with burns

Parkland formula	4 mL x body weight (kg) x %TBSA
	Half given over first 8 h, second half given over 16 h
Modified Brooke formula	2 mL x body weight (kg) x %TBSA
	Half given over first 8 h, second half given over 16 h

Operative Steps

Endotracheal Intubation

1. Ensure availability of equipment and intravenous access.
2. Administer sedative/paralytic.
3. Pre-oxygenate with bag mask.
4. Insert laryngoscope and attempt to identify view of the vocal cords, using suction or adjuncts such as video laryngoscope or gum bougie.
5. Intubate an appropriately sized endotracheal tube beyond the vocal cords.
6. Inflate balloon and confirm end-tidal CO_2.
7. Check bilateral breath sounds and obtain CXR.

Sequela

The bedside nurse and respiratory therapist are, respectively, concerned about the degree of circumferential burns across the upper arms and upper thorax. The respiratory therapist reports elevated airway resistance and the nurse reports bilateral lower arm/hand pallor and decreased pulses with worsening swelling.

What's the Working Diagnosis?

You are concerned about the constricting eschar causing compartment syndrome. You plan on escharotomy.

Operative Steps

Escharotomy

1. On the extremities, incise the complete thickness of the dermis in a longitudinal fashion on medial and lateral surfaces, extending from 1 cm proximal to 1 cm distal.
2. On the chest, incise the complete thickness of the dermis along bilateral anterior axillary lines with transverse incisions across mid-chest and subcostal region.
3. On the neck, incise the complete thickness of the dermis posterior and lateral to the sternocleidomastoid muscle.

Sequela

The patient maintains excellent urine output and is started on IV nutrition. The patient is stabilized and ready for early excision and grafting.

Operative Steps

Burn Excision

1. Ensure adequate resuscitative access, several units of crossed blood, and operating room warming.
2. Plan to excise largest areas first up to a maximum of 40% TBSA at any given time.
3. Perform tangential excision to maximize dermal preservation down to healthy bleeding tissue.
4. Minimize excessive blood loss with tourniquet use, topical hemostatics, use of tumescent epinephrine, and rapid coverage of the excised wound.
5. Apply autograft, allograft, temporary moist dressings with topical ointments (silver sulfadiazine, mafenide acetate, bacitracin, etc.), or biologics.

Sequela

You are able to graft the chest and abdomen but run out of available donor sites for the arms, so you opt to temporize the arms with frequent dressing changes with silver sulfadiazine. After several days of dressing changes, the bedside nurse inquires why the skin appears discolored and if they should be concerned about the dropping blood cell counts.

What's the Diagnosis?

You describe the discoloration and cytopenias are likely side effects of the silver sulfadiazine. You plan on re-harvesting split thickness skin grafts (STSG) to cover the remaining wounds as soon as the donor sites heal.

Operative Steps

Split Thickness Skin Grafting

1. Confirm that the recipient wound bed has healthy granulation tissue with no sign of necrosis or infection.
2. Select a donor site that has a large flat surface area such as abdomen, thighs, or the buttocks (or scalp in children).
3. Set the dermatome to a uniform desired thickness (0.15 to 0.60 mm).
4. Mesh the graft to cover a larger surface area but not over joints or cosmetic areas.
5. Secure with staples, sutures, sealants, vacuum dressing, etc.
6. Evaluate for graft take in 3–5 days.

Sequela

You take down your covering dressings to evaluate for graft take. You notice that parts of the STSG appear to be lifting up and appear not perfused.

What's Your Next Step?

You opt to debride the portions that have failed and protect with regular moist dressing changes to allow reepithelialization or until you are able to attempt regrafting.

Case Scenario

Your next incoming trauma patient is a 58-year-old obese gentleman with cardiovascular comorbidities who sustained a stab wound to the left chest. The first responders en route report that the patient is in extremis. They have intubated and given TXA and two liters of crystalloid. They are currently transfusing uncrossed blood. By the time they arrive, they are performing chest compressions.

What's the Working Diagnosis?

Anything in the box may be injured. You are concerned about cardiac, lung, or great vessel injury.

What's Your Next Step?

You confirm airway, ventilation, and adequate IV access. You immediately note that there are no breath sounds on the left side.

What's the Working Diagnosis?

You are concerned about mainstem intubation or pneumothorax. Retracting the endotracheal tube slightly makes no improvement. You perform a finger thoracotomy and there is immediate decompression of air. You place a definitive tube thoracostomy. The team reports ROSC. After completing your primary and secondary survey with findings of no additional injury, you place the patient in the ICU.

The Scenario Changes

Suppose the patient does not improve with tube thoracostomy; rather the tube begins draining large volumes of bright red blood. The patient still has not recovered ROSC. You opt to perform emergency resuscitative thoracotomy on the left.

Operative Steps

Resuscitative Thoracotomy

1. Elevate ipsilateral arm and splash Betadine prep if available.
2. Incise the chest along the fifth intercostal space from contralateral sternum to the axilla down to rib periosteum.
3. Divide the intercostal muscles and insert the Finochietto rib spreader with prongs facing medial.
4. Incise pericardium anterior and parallel to the phrenic nerve to evacuate any hemopericardium (Fig. 1.2).
5. Other maneuvers that may be accomplished within the chest: elevate and rotate the lobe if major lung bleeding is identified, cross-clamp the thoracic aorta if proximal control is needed, or perform cardiac massage between two hands.

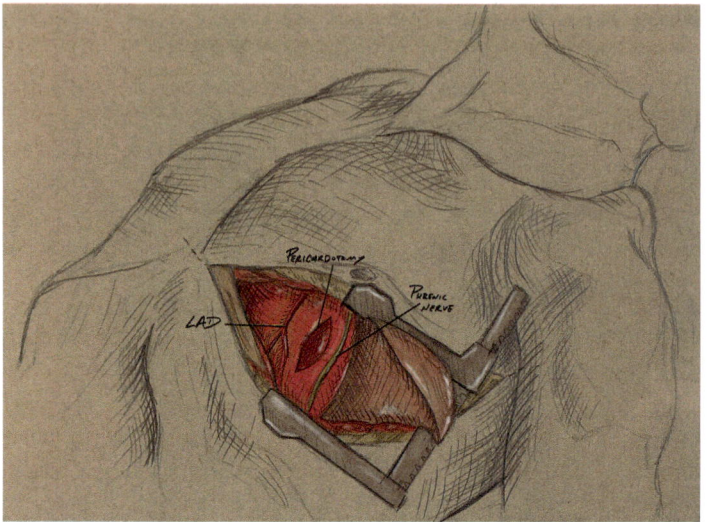

Fig. 1.2   Pericardiotomy during resuscitative thoracotomy

Sequela

The patient recovers hemodynamically and eventually is able to be extubated but has not recovered appropriate mental status. Workup confirms anoxic brain injury. Family has been contacted and they wish to proceed with full supportive measures. The ICU team has inquired about surgical long-term feeding access. The patient has been tolerating nasoenteric tube feeds.

Operative Steps

Percutaneous Endoscopic Gastrostomy

1. Introduce the scope into the mouth after positioning supine with bite block in place and intubate the esophagus.
2. Evaluate for abnormalities en route to the stomach.
3. Insufflate the stomach.

4. Observe for 1:1 ballottement and transillumination to select an optimal site of gastrostomy placement at least two fingerbreadths distal to the rib.
5. Ensure pylorus is at a distance to avoid iatrogenic outlet obstruction from the balloon.
6. Aspirate air and observe for bubbles and simultaneous intragastric visualization of the needle.
7. Place the gastrostomy tube via push or pull technique.
8. Confirm easy rotation of the final tube balloon or bumper.
9. Secure and document depth of insertion.
10. Leave to gravity drainage; allow use for meds or feeds after a period of 6–24 h.

Sequela

While performing the endoscopy, you are unable to obtain a safe site for percutaneous placement. You abort the procedure and return the patient to the unit. You speak with family about laparoscopic, possible open, gastrostomy placement. The family consents.

Operative Steps

Laparoscopic Gastrostomy

1. Position the patient supine with arms tucked.
2. Access and insufflate the peritoneal cavity.
3. Place a camera port at or above the umbilicus; introduce a grasper through the future gastrostomy site.
4. Grasp the stomach's anterior surface at the anticipated gastrotomy.
5. Suture from stomach to abdominal wall on either side of the gastrotomy.
6. Under direct visualization, remove the grasper and introduce a needle into the stomach, followed by wire insertion, dilation, and gastrostomy tube insertion and balloon inflation.
7. Secure the sutures, desufflate the abdomen, and close the port site.

Open Gastrostomy

1. Perform supraumbilical midline laparotomy.
2. Select a point on the anterior stomach which will easily reach the abdominal wall and the selected gastrostomy tube site.
3. Place two purse-string sutures encircling the planned tube insertion on the stomach wall.
4. Make a skin incision and gastrotomy within the purse-string and pass the gastrostomy tube and inflate the balloon.
5. Tie down the purse-string sutures, securing the outer to the abdominal wall.
6. Secure the stomach at the three other quadrants to the abdominal wall.
7. Close the abdomen.

Additional Reading

1. Eastern Association for the Surgery of Trauma. Practice Management Guidelines. https://www.east.org/education-resources/practice-management-guidelines. 2024. Accessed 30 Dec 2024.
2. Ley D, Austin K, Wilson KA, Saha S. Tutorial on adult enteral tube feeding: indications, placement, removal, complications, and ethics. JPEN J Parenter Enteral Nutr. 2023;47(5):677–85. https://doi.org/10.1002/jpen.2510. Epub 2023 May 23. PMID: 37122159.
3. Sinz E, Navarro K. ACLS for experienced providers: manual and resource text. Dallas: American Heart Association; 2017.
4. Taylor BC, Triplet JJ, Wells M. Split-thickness skin grafting: a primer for Orthopaedic surgeons. J Am Acad Orthop Surg. 2021;29(20):855–61. https://doi.org/10.5435/JAAOS-D-20-01389. PMID: 34547758.
5. Walker B, Axtell AL. Management of Tracheoesophageal Fistula and Tracheoinnominate Fistula. Thorac Surg Clin. 2025;35(1):73–81. https://doi.org/10.1016/j.thorsurg.2024.07.006. Epub 2024 Aug 13. PMID: 39515897.
6. Western Trauma Association. Western Trauma Association Algorithms. http://westerntrauma.org/algorithms.php. 2024. Accessed 30 Dec 2024.
7. Zhang L, Labib A, Hughes PG. Escharotomy. 2023 Aug 14. In: StatPearls [Internet]. Treasure Island (FL): StatPearls Publishing. 2024. PMID: 29489153.

Hepatobiliary

Case Scenario

You are called to see a 48-year-old obese woman who presented to the emergency room with acute onset of right upper quadrant pain of four hours, preceded by a large dinner and accompanied by nausea and vomiting. She has had similar episodes in the past after consuming fatty meals. A right upper quadrant ultrasound reveals a distended gallbladder with gallstones, pericholecystic fluid, thickened gallbladder wall, and a common bile duct of 1.5 cm diameter. Her bloodwork is notable for a serum white blood cell count of 14×10^9/L and a serum total bilirubin of 2.1 mg/dL. She is tender in the epigastrium but afebrile and hemodynamically normal.

What's the Working Diagnosis?

You are concerned about acute cholecystitis with choledocholithiasis. The differential includes biliary colic, symptomatic cholelithiasis, ascending cholangitis, or choledochal cyst.

What's Your Treatment Plan?

You admit the patient nil per os, start intravenous antibiotics, and consult gastroenterology for endoscopic retrograde cholangio-pancreatography to evaluate and clear any common duct stones. Unfortunately, gastroenterology is not available.

You consent the patient for laparoscopic cholecystectomy with intraoperative cholangiography and possible common bile duct exploration.

Operative Steps

Laparoscopic Cholecystectomy

1. Insufflate the abdomen and place two lateral ports subcostal in the right upper quadrant, a supraumbilical port, and a subxiphoid port (Fig. 2.1).
2. Elevate the fundus toward the diaphragm and retract laterally.
3. Dissect out the cystic artery and duct, achieving the critical view of safety prior to dividing the structures.
4. Perform intraoperative cholangiography at this time if indicated.
5. Divide the cystic artery and duct and free the specimen from the cystic plate.
6. Ensure hemostasis; aspirate any spilled stones or bile; desufflate and close the abdomen including the fascia for any port sites larger than 8 mm.

Intraoperative Cholangiogram (Table 2.1)

1. Apply a cholangiography clamp across the infundibulum and advance the needle and catheter into the cystic duct.
2. Obtain fluoroscopic image after injecting a contrast load.
3. Confirm passage of contrast proximally into the biliary tree and distally into the duodenum.

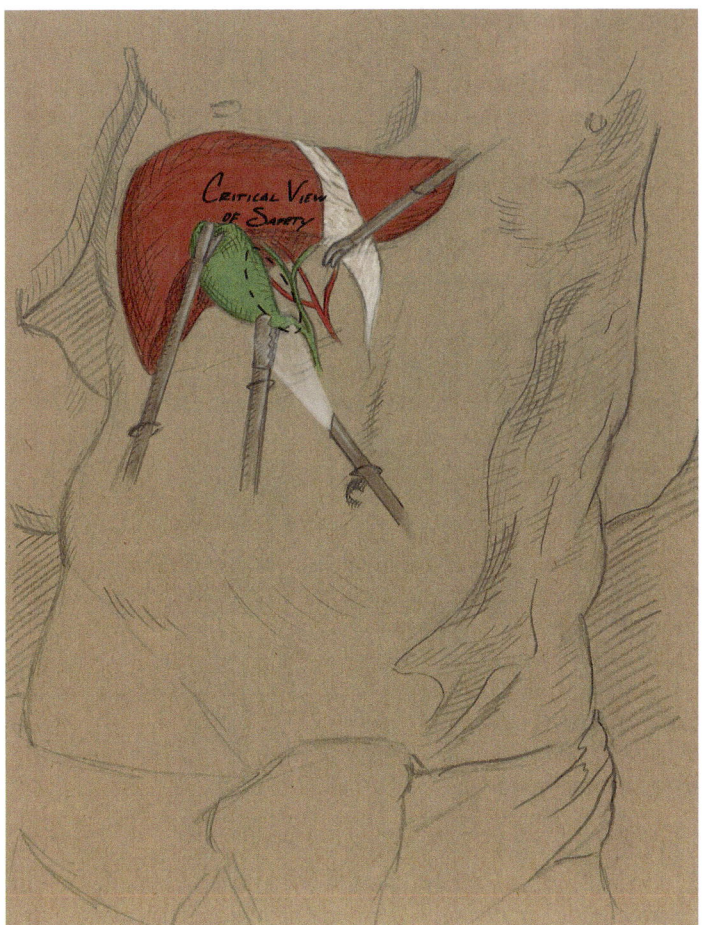

Fig. 2.1 Laparoscopic cholecystectomy port sites and instrumentation at the critical view of safety

Table 2.1 Alternative techniques for intraoperative cholangiography

Divide the cystic duct after clipping the distal stump and feed a catheter into the proximal stump and secure with a clip
Insert a long needle directly into the common bile duct
Utilize a choledochoscope via the cystic duct

Open Cholecystectomy

1. Enter the abdominal cavity via a curved transverse right sub-costal incision, dividing the fascia and muscle.
2. Dissect free the gallbladder from the cystic plate using a dome-down approach.
3. Dissect out the cystic artery and duct, achieving the critical view of safety prior to dividing the structures.
4. Perform intraoperative cholangiography at this time if indicated.
5. Divide the cystic artery and duct and pass off the specimen.
6. Ensure hemostasis, aspirate any spilled stones or bile, and close the abdominal wall in layers using running suture.

Sequela

The cholecystectomy is completed without difficulty and the cholangiogram reveals an impacted stone. You proceed with attempts at clearing the duct.

Operative Steps

Bile Duct Clearance

1. Flush with saline.
2. Flush again with saline 30–60 seconds after anesthesia administers 1 mg of glucagon. This can be repeated a second time.
3. If unable to flush, divide and dilate the cystic duct and retrieve the stone using a balloon catheter (7 Fr) or a basket.
4. Perform a completion cholangiogram to confirm passage of contrast proximally into biliary tree and distally into duodenum.
5. If continued attempts to clear the duct fail, perform a bile duct exploration.

Laparoscopic Common Bile Duct Exploration

1. Create an additional subcostal port and insert a choledocho-scope into the cystic duct after dividing the duct, dilating the duct, and clearing the cystic duct of stones.
2. If unable to insert into the cystic duct, use an endoscopic scal-pel to incise the anterior surface of the common bile duct below the insertion of the cystic duct.
3. Milk out, flush, or retrieve any stones.
4. Using the choledochoscope, visually confirm that the entirety of the duct is cleared of stones.
5. Close the choledochotomy over a T-tube using continuous absorbable running suture. If the cystic duct was used as the insertion point, this may be ligated with an endoloop.
6. Remove the T-tube if a tube study in 1–2 weeks reveals a pat-ent biliary system and the patient experiences no symptoms upon tube clamping.

Open Common Bile Duct Exploration

1. Enter the abdominal cavity via a curved transverse subcostal incision, dividing the fascia and muscle.
2. Using a retractor system, retract liver superiorly and intestines inferiorly.
3. Open up the hepatoduodenal ligament to identify the common bile duct.
4. Perform a longitudinal 1 cm choledochotomy at the midpor-tion of the common duct.
5. Milk out, flush, or retrieve stones.
6. Using the choledochoscope, visually confirm that the entirety of the duct is cleared of stones.
7. Close the choledochotomy over a T-tube using continuous absorbable running suture.
8. Close the incision in layers.
9. Remove the T-tube if a tube study in 1–2 weeks reveals a pat-ent biliary system and the patient experiences no symptoms upon tube clamping.

Sequela

You successfully clear the stone laparoscopically without needing to explore the duct, and a completion cholangiogram reveals passage of contrast into the biliary tree and into the duodenum. The patient recovers well and goes home. She returns five days later to the emergency room with a similar presentation of acute right upper quadrant pain and low-grade fevers. Bloodwork reveals mild leukocytosis and an elevated total bilirubin. A computed tomography (CT) scan reveals a fluid collection in the gallbladder fossa.

What's the Working Diagnosis?

You are concerned about a bile leak leading to formation of a biloma (Table 2.2).

Table 2.2 Differential diagnosis of a post-cholecystectomy fluid collection

Seroma
Organ space surgical site infection without bile leak
Perforated appendicitis
Perforated peptic ulcer disease
Perforated right-sided diverticulitis

What's Your Treatment Plan?

You decide to admit the patient nil per os, start intravenous antibiotics, and consult interventional radiology to place a percutaneous drainage catheter into the presumptive biloma. You also consult gastroenterology for endoscopic retrograde cholangiopancreatography to identify the source of the bile leak and potentially stent the common bile duct.

A percutaneous drainage catheter is placed which drains fluid consistent with bile. The gastroenterologist identifies a bile leak occurring just distal to the junction of the right and left hepatic ducts. You consent the patient for exploratory laparotomy with hepaticojejunostomy.

Operative Steps

Hepaticojejunostomy

1. Enter the abdominal cavity via a midline celiotomy or curved subcostal incision.
2. Using a retractor system, retract liver superiorly and intestines inferiorly.
3. Perform a Kocher maneuver (or, described alternatively, a "lateral to medial mobilization of the duodenum").
4. Open up the hepatoduodenal ligament to identify the common hepatic duct and site of leak.
5. Debride proximal and distal biliary duct ends to viable tissue and ligate the distal stump.
6. Elevate the transverse mesocolon to identify the ligament of Treitz.
7. Perform stapled transection of the small bowel 35 cm distal to the ligament to create a Roux-en-Y jejunal limb or select a freely mobile loop of jejunum to pass antecolic. If creating Roux-en-Y anatomy, select a more distal segment to create the enteroenterostomy to restore the patient's intestinal continuity and close the mesenteric defects.

8. Create a hepaticojejunostomy using fine monofilament suture (5–0 or smaller) between the proximal hepatic duct stump and an enterotomy made in the jejunum limb or loop in a tension-free manner.
9. Ensure hemostasis, consider omental flap and wide drainage, and close the abdominal wall in layers.

The Scenario Changes

Suppose the patient did not experience a bile leak and returns instead to your office three weeks after your successful laparoscopic cholecystectomy. On final pathology, the specimen revealed an incidental finding of gallbladder adenocarcinoma extending to the muscularis of the specimen wall. The bile duct margin is negative.

What's the Working Diagnosis?

You are concerned about a T1b gallbladder cancer.

What's Your Treatment Plan?

You discuss the need for an oncologic resection pending staging scans and multidisciplinary tumor board discussion. Tumor markers including carcinoembryonic antigen (CEA) and cancer antigen 19–9 (CA 19–9) and repeat bloodwork are sent. Presuming the patient is an operative candidate, you consent the patient for partial hepatectomy of segment IVb/V and portal lymphadenectomy.

Operative Steps

Completion Radical Resection for T1b Gallbladder Cancer

1. Discuss with anesthesiology the need to minimize volume resuscitation to manage blood loss.
2. Enter the abdominal cavity via a midline celiotomy or curved subcostal incision (alternatives include Chevron, modified Chevron "Mercedes-Benz," modified Makuuchi, etc.).
3. Using a retractor system, retract the ribcage superiorly and intestines inferiorly.
4. Consider means of vascular control (Table 2.3).
5. Utilize a technique of choice of parenchymal transection (Table 2.4) to take a 2 cm margin from segments IVb and V, which is determined with the aid of frozen section.
6. Ensure hemostasis with consideration for application of hemostatic agents, consider wide drainage, and close the abdomen in layers.

Table 2.3 Methods of vascular control for liver resection

Perform a portal triad clamp (Pringle maneuver) manually, with a Rummel tourniquet, with a vascular clamp, etc., continuously or intermittently
Perform total hepatic vascular occlusion by fully mobilizing the liver and controlling the portal triad plus the infrahepatic and suprahepatic IVC, or just the portal triad and extrahepatic hepatic veins to preserve caval flow
Ligate the feeding hepatic pedicle (left, right, segment, etc.)

Table 2.4 Techniques for hepatic parenchymal transection

Crush clamp
Ultrasonic aspirator (i.e., Cavitron, harmonic scalpel)
Sealing device (i.e., LigaSure)
Water-jet dissector
Vascular staplers

Sequela

The patient undergoes a successful operation with negative margins and proceeds to adjuvant chemotherapy. You plan to surveil the patient with repeat imaging every six months for two years with repeat tumor markers as clinically indicated.

Case Scenario

You are called to see a 63-year-old man in the emergency room for progressive worsening right upper quadrant pain associated with intermittent fevers and chills. The patient recently returned from a business trip in Southeast Asia. His medical history includes type 2 diabetes on insulin, former alcoholism, and a recent cholecystectomy. He has a leukocytosis and transaminitis. His total bilirubin is top normal. His heart rate is 100 bpm and his temperature is 38.3 C. He is tender in the right upper quadrant to palpation.

What's the Working Diagnosis?

You are concerned about a hepatic infection, which may be hepatitis, hepatic abscess (pyogenic, amebic, or parasitic), or cholangitis. Other possibilities include a retained common bile duct stone after his recent cholecystectomy or a malignancy.

What's Your Next Step?

You obtain additional bloodwork including hepatitis panel, blood cultures, serologic tests, and cross-sectional imaging. You initiate the patient on broad-spectrum antibiotics. The serologic tests return positive for *Entamoeba histolytica*. Cross-sectional imaging reveals a 4 cm hepatic lesion consistent with abscess.

What's Your Treatment Plan?

You treat with metronidazole for 5–10 days.

The Scenario Changes

Instead of presenting acutely, this patient reports during a clinic visit that he has been experiencing progressive right upper quadrant discomfort. Radiographic imaging demonstrated a large hepatic cyst. Serologic tests are positive for *Echinococcus granulosus*.

What's Your Treatment Plan?

You treat with albendazole for 1–3 months. You consider consultation with radiology and hepatology for a puncture, aspiration, injection, and re-aspiration procedure if indicated.

The Scenario Changes

Instead of returning from a recent trip to Southeast Asia, this patient has returned from a recent bout of perforated appendicitis. The perforation was found intraoperatively and the appendix had been removed. The patient had been discharged from the hospital on postoperative day four. It is now postoperative day eight. He reports worsening fevers and right upper abdominal pain. He has a neutrophilic leukocytosis with a CT scan revealing a 5 cm hepatic abscess.

What's the Working Diagnosis?

You are concerned about a pyogenic liver abscess secondary to perforated appendicitis.

What's Your Treatment Plan?

In addition to hospital admission and broad-spectrum antibiotics, you consult interventional radiology for percutaneous drainage and ask for culture of the aspirate to help narrow antibiotic therapy.

The radiologist indicates that the abscess is too posterior to adequately approach percutaneously and insists you perform surgical drainage.

Operative Steps

Laparoscopic Hepatic Abscess Drainage

1. Place a camera and two or more working ports along cholecystectomy port sites (in cases of pyogenic liver abscess of biliary origin, it may be prudent to remove the gallbladder in the same case).
2. Use a suction irrigator to bluntly penetrate into the abscess cavity and aspirate pus.
3. Copiously irrigate both the abscess cavity and the abdominal cavity.
4. Unroof the abscess cavity where feasible and leave a surgical drain.

Sequela

Intraoperative cultures speciate and guide your antibiotic therapy. The patient clinically improves and is discharged from the hospital. At follow-up, the drain has minimal output and the abscess has resolved on repeat radiographic imaging, after which the drain is removed.

Case Scenario

You are seeing a 74-year-old woman in your office in referral for a 3 cm liver lesion found on imaging performed during an admission for a motor vehicle collision. She is otherwise well and sustained no significant injuries. She denies any abnormal symptoms. She is unaware of any relevant family history. She has had negative colonoscopies throughout her life. You have not yet received access to the CT scan or any bloodwork, but the patient recalls the lesion was "hyperenhancing." Her physical exam is unremarkable.

What's the Working Diagnosis?

You are concerned for a hepatic malignancy (Table 2.5).

Table 2.5 Differential diagnosis of liver lesions

Cystic lesions:
Simple cyst
Infectious
Malignancy
Solid lesions:
Hypervascular:
Benign: Focal nodular hyperplasia, hemangioma, adenoma
Malignant: Hepatocellular carcinoma, cholangiocarcinoma, neuroendocrine
Hypovascular:
Metastases

What's Your Next Step?

You obtain multiphase contrast CT if it was not already performed as well as complete metabolic panel, blood count, hepatitis panel, and tumor markers including alpha-fetoprotein (AFP), CA 19–9, and CEA. The bloodwork is largely unrevealing, but the radiographic interpretation describes a single 3 cm tumor in Couinaud segment III suspicious for hepatocellular carcinoma (HCC) in a background of mild cirrhosis. Due to intervening bowel, the interventional radiologist is unwilling to percutaneously access the lesion for diagnostic biopsy.

What's the Treatment Plan?

After discussing the patient case in a multidisciplinary tumor board, you consent the patient for diagnostic laparoscopy, laparoscopic ultrasound-guided biopsy, and possible left lateral segmentectomy if biopsy is confirmatory of HCC and there are no other contraindications to proceeding with resection, including preoperative assessment of the functional liver remnant.

The patient asks you under what circumstances could she receive a liver transplant instead. You advise her that transplant eligibility is based on certain criteria (Table 2.6) specified by organizations such as the United Network for Organ Sharing (UNOS).

Table 2.6 UNOS criteria for liver transplant for HCC

AFP <1000 ng/mL
1 tumor with diameter 2–5 cm
2–3 tumors each with diameter 1–3 cm
No macrovascular involvement
No extrahepatic disease
Surgically unresectable due to location, degree of cirrhosis, presence of portal hypertension, inadequate liver remnant

Operative Steps

Laparoscopic Liver Biopsy

1. Place a camera and two or more working 5 mm ports in the epigastric/subcostal region (these may be positioned suitable for proceeding with resection, so along right subcostal if resecting right segments and along bilateral subcostal if approaching the left).
2. Identify the lesion visually, by instrument palpation, or with laparoscopic ultrasound.
3. Obtain a wedge excision or perform core needle biopsy under visual or ultrasound guidance and send the specimen for pathology (frozen or permanent based on the situation).
4. Ensure hemostasis with pressure, electrocautery, and/or hemostatic agents.

> **Operative Pearl**
>
> Laparoscopic ultrasound works better under submersion with saline.

The pathologist reports findings consistent with HCC on the frozen section. You proceed as planned with resection.

Operative Steps

Laparoscopic Hepatic Resection

1. If not already done, obtain vascular control (Table 2.3).
2. Delineate border of the resection segment/section using intraoperative ultrasound.
3. Use preferred choice of parenchymal transection (Table 2.4) and ligate biliary radicals and large vessels as they are encountered.
4. Ensure adequate hemostasis and widely drain.

Sequela

Postoperatively, the patient experiences worsening fluid overload, oliguria, confusion, and oxygen requirement. Bloodwork demonstrates an elevated creatinine.

What's the Working Diagnosis?

Although a simple acute kidney injury (AKI) can occur at any time after major abdominal surgery, its occurrence following any hepatic resection or in the presence of liver disease warrants consideration for hepatorenal syndrome.

What's the Treatment Plan?

Given the tenuous respiratory status, you cautiously administer crystalloid/colloid resuscitation and add on vasoconstrictors to promote renal perfusion if no response to simple resuscitation. You consult hepatology and nephrology for their assistance.

Additional Reading

1. Aragon RJ, Solomon NL. Techniques of hepatic resection. J Gastrointest Oncol. 2012;3(1):28–40. https://doi.org/10.3978/j.issn.2078-6891.2012.006. PMID: 22811867; PMCID: PMC3397635.
2. Heimbach JK. Evolution of liver transplant selection criteria and U.S. allocation policy for patients with hepatocellular carcinoma. Semin Liver Dis. 2020;40(4):358–64. https://doi.org/10.1055/s-0040-1709492. Epub 2020 Sep 17. PMID: 32942324.
3. Jackson PG, Evans SRT. Biliary system. In: Townsend CM, Daniel Beauchamp R, Mark Evers B, Mattox KL, Christopher F, editors. Sabiston textbook of surgery: the biological basis of modern surgical practice. Philadelphia: Elsevier; 2017. p. 1482–519.
4. Mownah OA, Aroori S. The Pringle maneuver in the modern era: A review of techniques for hepatic inflow occlusion in minimally invasive liver resection. Ann Hepatobiliary Pancreat Surg. 2023;27(2):131–40. https://

doi.org/10.14701/ahbps.22-109. Epub 2023 Mar 6. PMID: 36872860; PMCID: PMC10201059.

5. National Comprehensive Cancer Network. Biliary tract cancers. In: NCCN clinical practice guidelines in oncology; 2024. https://www.nccn.org/professionals/physician_gls/pdf/btc.pdf. Accessed 30 Dec 2024.

6. National Comprehensive Cancer Network. Hepatocellular Carcinoma. In: NCCN clinical practice guidelines in oncology; 2024. https://www.nccn.org/professionals/physician_gls/pdf/hcc.pdf. Accessed 30 Dec 2024.

7. Pisano M, Allievi N, Gurusamy K, Borzellino G, Cimbanassi S, Boerna D, Coccolini F, Tufo A, Di Martino M, Leung J, Sartelli M, Ceresoli M, Maier RV, Poiasina E, De Angelis N, Magnone S, Fugazzola P, Paolillo C, Coimbra R, Di Saverio S, De Simone B, Weber DG, Sakakushev BE, Lucianetti A, Kirkpatrick AW, Fraga GP, Wani I, Biffl WL, Chiara O, Abu-Zidan F, Moore EE, Leppäniemi A, Kluger Y, Catena F, Ansaloni L. 2020 World society of emergency surgery updated guidelines for the diagnosis and treatment of acute calculus cholecystitis. World J Emerg Surg. 2020;15(1):61. https://doi.org/10.1186/s13017-020-00336-x. PMID: 33153472; PMCID: PMC7643471.

8. Roediger R, Lisker-Melman M. Pyogenic and amebic infections of the liver. Gastroenterol Clin N Am. 2020;49(2):361–77. https://doi.org/10.1016/j.gtc.2020.01.013. PMID: 32389368.

9. Simonetto DA, Gines P, Kamath PS. Hepatorenal syndrome: pathophysiology, diagnosis, and management. BMJ. 2020;14(370):m2687. https://doi.org/10.1136/bmj.m2687. PMID: 32928750.

Foregut

3

Case Scenario

A 62-year-old man presents for referral for persistent gastro-esophageal reflux symptoms. He has had symptoms of heartburn and regurgitation in addition to a chronic cough. This has persisted despite trialing several proton pump inhibitors. He has never had endoscopic evaluation. He denies chest pain. His family history is negative.

What's Your Next Step?

In addition to an updated set of bloodwork, you plan on performing an upper endoscopy as well as obtaining esophageal manometry.

Operative Steps

Upper Endoscopy

1. Position the patient in left lateral decubitus or supine if proceeding under monitored anesthesia care versus general anesthesia.
2. Protect dentition with a bite block and intubate the esophagus.

© The Author(s), under exclusive license to Springer Nature Switzerland AG 2025
S. Hao et al., *General Surgery Boards Case-Based Review*,
https://doi.org/10.1007/978-3-031-85631-0_3

3. Traverse the esophagus keeping the lumen centered and noting landmarks such as the Z line as well as possible anomalies such as tumors, strictures, or mucosal changes.
4. Proceed through the stomach and intubate the pylorus to evaluate the first portion of the duodenum.
5. Retract back into the stomach and retroflex to view the hiatus.
6. Desufflate while retracting the scope to end the procedure.

You identify longitudinal streaks of abnormal mucosa suggestive of Barrett's. Four quadrant biopsies of the mucosa are consistent with intestinal metaplasia. There are no ulcers or strictures. Antral biopsies are negative for *H. pylori*. The manometry results indicate a dysfunctioning lower esophageal sphincter but normal esophageal motility.

What's the Treatment Plan?

You counsel the patient on dietary and lifestyle changes in addition to combination therapy with histamine H2-receptor antagonists, proton pump inhibitors, and antacids. You plan on repeat endoscopic and clinical evaluation in 6 months.

Sequela

At repeat evaluation, there are now superficial erosions in the esophageal lining, and the patient reports no improvement in symptoms. You discuss proceeding with an antireflux procedure.

Operative Steps

Laparoscopic Nissen Fundoplication (Fig. 3.1)

1. Place four or five ports across the upper abdomen after insufflation.

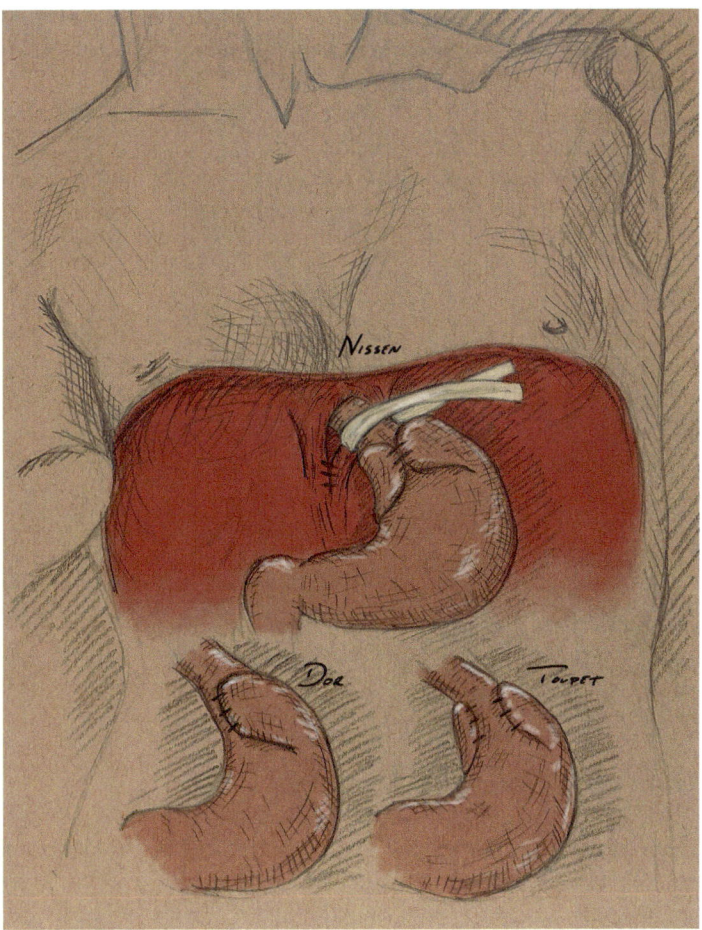

Fig. 3.1 Key steps of the Nissen fundoplication with final configurations of the Dor and Toupet fundoplications

2. Divide the lesser omentum up to and exposing the left crus, avoiding the anterior vagus nerve.
3. Divide short gastric vessels to free the greater curvature of the stomach.

4. Suture close the crura if there is also a hiatal hernia component, with a Penrose looped around the gastroesophageal junction as needed for retraction.
5. Pull the fundus posteriorly from left to right and slide back and forth in the shoeshine maneuver.
6. After anesthesia inserts a bougie dilator into the lumen, place interrupted sutures to secure the wrapped fundus to itself.

Sequela

Postoperatively, the patient is able to advance their diet with a significant improvement in reflux symptoms at their postoperative office visit. You plan to continue annual endoscopic surveillance of their Barrett's disease.

The Scenario Changes

Postoperatively, the patient experiences tachycardia with vague upper abdominal discomfort. Blood pressure is within normal limits.

What's the Working Diagnosis?

Tachycardia after any gastric surgery warrants consideration for possible leak or perforation. You make the patient nil per os, initiate resuscitation, and obtain an abdominal CT with oral contrast.

CT reveals small contained gastric perforation near the fundoplication.

What's Your Next Step?

You carefully and personally place a nasogastric decompression tube, keep the patient nil per os, consider initiation of parenteral nutrition, and initiate antibiotic coverage. The patient wants to know what would happen if the leak worsens. You advise in that situation, you would take the patient back to the operating room, obtain source control, attempt to repair and/or patch the leak, and widely drain.

Case Scenario

You are asked to consult on a 77-year-old woman with symptomatic anemia from a stomach mass (Table 3.1). Endoscopic workup by the gastroenterologist revealed a 3 cm submucosal tumor in the fundus of the stomach. Preliminary pathology from biopsies report spindle cells.

Table 3.1 Differential diagnosis of a stomach mass

Gastric adenocarcinoma
Gastric lymphoma
GIST
Sarcoma
Lipoma
Neuroendocrine tumor
Intramural hematoma

What's the Working Diagnosis?

A spindle cell submucosal tumor in the GI tract is most likely a gastrointestinal stromal tumor (GIST).

What's the Treatment Plan?

You discuss proceeding with surgical resection to negative margins.

Operative Steps

Wedge Gastrectomy

1. Access the abdomen open or laparoscopically and identify the tumor.
2. Open the lesser sac to evaluate the posterior surface of the stomach.
3. Survey the abdominal cavity for peritoneal metastases.
4. Staple or transect a portion of the stomach wall to include the tumor in its entirety.
5. Suture in two layers if stapled resection was not used.
6. Consider omental patch coverage.
7. Leave a nasogastric tube in place for decompression.

Sequela

Postoperatively, the patient experiences a massive myocardial infarction with significant hemodynamic collapse. The patient is intubated and resuscitated and taken to the cardiac ICU for further care. You are called to evaluate worsening abdominal distension. The ICU team reports elevated peak airway pressures and an elevated bladder pressure despite paralysis. The patient also has a worsening acute kidney injury with progressive oliguria.

What's the Working Diagnosis?

You are concerned about abdominal compartment syndrome given the combination of intra-abdominal hypertension along with organ failure and dysfunction.

What's the Treatment Plan?

You consent family and proceed with decompressive laparotomy with temporary abdominal closure, with plans to attempt fascial closure as early as feasible.

Sequela

The patient recovers and is able to be discharged to a facility. The final pathology confirms the GIST was completely resected as well as the presence of a KIT mutation suggesting sensitivity to adjuvant treatment. You refer the patient to an oncologist to begin imatinib. You plan to surveil the patient every six months for five years with repeat exams and cross-sectional imaging.

Case Scenario

You are called to see a 57-year-old man who was admitted to the ICU for shock. He had presented hours earlier with large-volume hematemesis. The patient is currently awake and alert. He vomited several times prior to presentation and reports a maroon-colored vomitus. He is not aware of any melena. He has never had surgery. He has been self-medicating with daily ibuprofen for a sprained ankle sustained six months prior, in addition to his daily aspirin 325 mg. He has already received two liters of normal saline and two units of blood for his hypotension, tachycardia, and hemoglobin of 5.7 g/dL. Gastroenterologists are unavailable. He is tender in the epigastrium and appears pale and uncomfortable, and his current vitals are heart rate of 105 bpm, cuff blood pressure of 100/54 mmHg, and respiratory rate of 26.

What's the Working Diagnosis?

You are concerned about an upper GI bleed, likely from a peptic ulcer in the setting of nonsteroidal anti-inflammatory drug (NSAID) use. Your differential also includes Mallory-Weiss tear, a Dieulafoy lesion, gastroesophageal varices, or a marginal ulcer in the setting of relevant prior surgical history.

What's Your Treatment Plan?

You send for additional bloodwork including repeat blood count, complete metabolic panel, and coagulation factor test. You request adequate intravenous access, invasive monitoring such as an arterial line and a central venous line, ongoing hemodynamic resuscitation, and correction of coagulopathy including platelet function in the setting of NSAIDs and of electrolyte abnormalities. You consent the patient for endoscopy to be performed within 24 h of patient presentation.

On endoscopic evaluation, you find an actively bleeding ulcer in the antrum of the stomach.

You treat the bleeding ulcer with epinephrine successfully (Table 3.2).

Table 3.2 Endoscopic interventions for bleeding lesions

Thermal coagulation
Injection of epinephrine
Clip application
Banding

Sequela

The patient again decompensates with dropping hemoglobin, bloody stools and nasogastric output, and hemodynamic instability. You plan to repeat your endoscopy.

On repeat endoscopy, the original antral ulcer is not bleeding. However, upon entering the duodenum, there is significant fresh blood impeding visualization. You are not able to visualize or treat a source of bleeding despite all attempts to lavage and inspect the mucosa.

What's the Treatment Plan?

You reach out to consult interventional radiology for angiographic identification and embolization of the bleeding, but they are not available. You opt to take the patient for surgical intervention on a presumptive bleeding peptic ulcer given the patient's instability.

Operative Steps

Duodenal Ulcer Surgery

1. Access the abdomen with a supraumbilical midline celiotomy.
2. Trace the stomach and identify the pylorus and first portion of the duodenum.
3. Incise the duodenum longitudinally on the anterior surface across the pylorus and onto the stomach.
4. Identify and oversew the ulcer superiorly, inferiorly, and medially.
5. Split the pylorus muscle and close transversely to widen the lumen (pyloroplasty).
6. Consider an omental patch and widely drain.

Truncal Vagotomy

1. Identify the left anterior and right posterior vagal trunks at the intra-abdominal esophagus.
2. Clip and resect a 2 cm segment of each trunk and send for pathology.

The Scenario Changes

Suppose it is not a duodenal ulcer but rather the antral ulcer that persistently bleeds despite endoscopic interventions. In the operating room, you are unable to cease the bleeding of the ulcer and opt to proceed with antrectomy (Fig. 3.2).

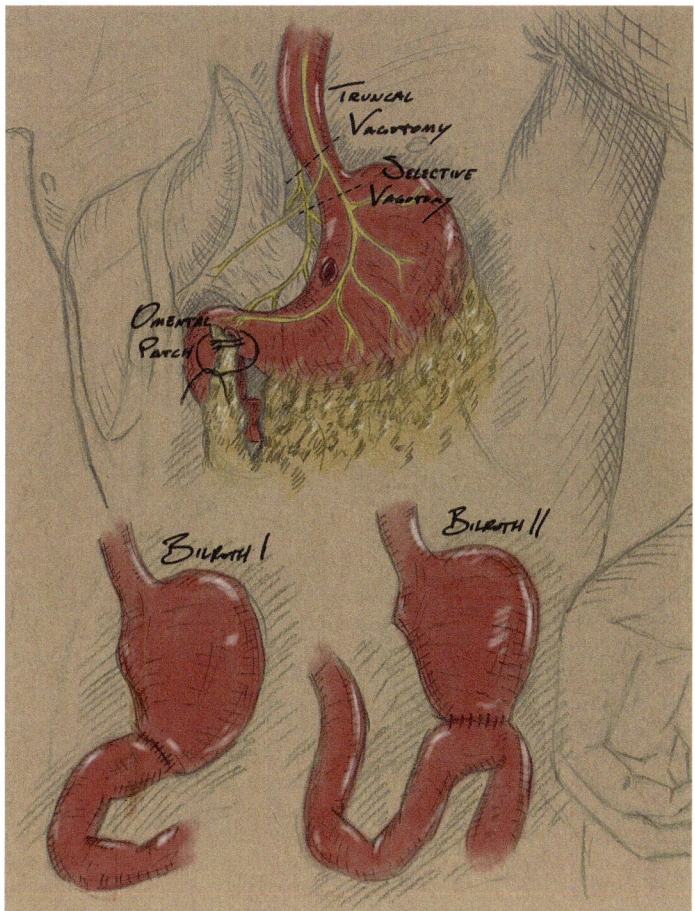

Fig. 3.2 Repair, acid control, and reconstruction in the treatment of gastro-duodenal ulcers

Operative Steps

Antrectomy with Reconstruction

1. Mobilize the attachments of the distal stomach to the lesser omentum and to the greater omentum.
2. Ligate the right gastroepiploic artery and the right gastric artery at the incisura.

3. Staple transect across the lower third of the stomach at the incisura.
4. Mobilize the duodenum and staple transect 2 cm beyond the pylorus.
5. Perform either a Billroth I or Billroth II gastrojejunostomy in either retrocolic or antecolic fashion.
6. Widely drain including consideration of a nasoenteric decompression tube.

Additional Reading

1. Imai TA, Soukiasian HJ. Management of Complications in Paraesophageal hernia repair. Thorac Surg Clin. 2019;29(4):351–8. https://doi.org/10.1016/j.thorsurg.2019.07.009. Epub 2019 Aug 30. PMID: 31564391.
2. Katz PO, Dunbar KB, Schnoll-Sussman FH, Greer KB, Yadlapati R, Spechler SJ. ACG clinical guideline for the diagnosis and Management of Gastroesophageal Reflux Disease. Am J Gastroenterol. 2022;117(1):27–56. https://doi.org/10.14309/ajg.0000000000001538. PMID: 34807007; PMCID: PMC8754510.
3. Kirkpatrick AW, Roberts DJ, De Waele J, Jaeschke R, Malbrain ML, De Keulenaer B, Duchesne J, Bjorck M, Leppaniemi A, Ejike JC, Sugrue M, Cheatham M, Ivatury R, Ball CG, Reintam Blaser A, Regli A, Balogh ZJ, D'Amours S, Debergh D, Kaplan M, Kimball E, Olvera C. Pediatric guidelines sub-committee for the world society of the abdominal compartment syndrome. intra-abdominal hypertension and the abdominal compartment syndrome: updated consensus definitions and clinical practice guidelines from the world society of the abdominal compartment syndrome. Intensive Care Med. 2013;39(7):1190–206. https://doi.org/10.1007/s00134-013-2906-z. Epub 2013 May 15. PMID: 23673399; PMCID: PMC3680657.
4. National Comprehensive Cancer Network. Gastrointestinal stromal tumors. In: NCCN clinical practice guidelines in oncology; 2024. https://www.nccn.org/professionals/physician_gls/pdf/gist.pdf. Accessed 30 Dec 2024.
5. Wang A, Yerxa J, Agarwal S, Turner MC, Schroder V, Youngwirth LM, Lagoo-Deenadayalan S, Pappas TN. Surgical management of peptic ulcer disease. Curr Probl Surg. 2020;57(2):100728. https://doi.org/10.1016/j.cpsurg.2019.100728. Epub 2020 Jan 7. PMID: 32138833.

Intestinal and Anorectal

4

Case Scenario

A 29-year-old female diagnosed with Crohn's disease at age 15 presents to the emergency room with nausea and vomiting associated with abdominal pain for three days. She has not been able to keep anything down. She was previously on biologic therapy with her disease in remission but due to insurance has not been able to receive her injection for the last six months. Her last colonoscopy was two years ago. She is tachycardic and normotensive. Her urine is concentrated. She has never had surgery before. An upright abdominal plain film reveals dilated loops of bowel with air fluid levels. She reports she was in the hospital twice in the last two months with bowel obstructions that resolved with conservative management. Her C-reactive protein (CRP) is mildly elevated.

What's the Working Diagnosis?

You are concerned for small bowel obstruction due to acute Crohn's flare.

What's Your Next Step?

You place a nasogastric tube and connect to low wall suction, start fluid resuscitation, and admit the patient to the hospital. You consult gastroenterology for consideration for steroid treatment for presumptive flare.

Sequela

The patient improves after resuscitation but her nasogastric tube continues to have high output. Gastroenterology obtains CT enterography which reveals mild terminal ileitis with fibrotic stricture in the proximal ileum.

What's the Treatment Plan?

You counsel the patient on the need for surgical exploration given that the stricture appears to be chronic fibrosis rather than acute inflammation.

Operative Steps

Small Bowel Resection

1. Identify segments of healthy bowel as points of proximal and distal transection.
2. Create a window in the mesentery and staple the bowel.
3. Transect the mesentery with tissue sealing device of choice.
4. Appose the remaining bowel and place securement sutures.
5. Create enterotomies at the staple lines and fire a staple load to create the common channel.
6. Close the common enterotomy with sutures or staples.

The Scenario Changes

In the operating room, you discover multiple segments of chronic strictures. You are concerned that the patient might be left with only 150 cm of small bowel if you were to resect all of the segments.

What's the Treatment Plan?

You evaluate each segment in consideration for stricturoplasty. You select the method of stricturoplasty based on length of the stricture.

Operative Steps

Heinecke-Mikulicz (up to 10 cm)

1. Create longitudinal enterotomy across length of stricture.
2. Close transversely with interrupted absorbable monofilament suture.

Finney Stricturoplasty (10–20 cm)

1. Incise a longitudinal enterotomy on the anti-mesenteric surface of the stricture.
2. Fold the bowel to appose the sides of the enterotomy.
3. Suture one end of the folded enterotomy to the other to create a side to side end to end common channel.

Michelassi Stricturoplasty (>20 cm)

1. Transect the length of strictured bowel into two equal halves.
2. Perform longitudinal enterotomies on the anti-mesenteric surface of the strictured segments.

3. Appose the halves of bowel in isoperistaltic fashion, partially dividing the mesentery to allow this position.
4. Suture the two large enterotomies with absorbable monofilament suture to create a single common channel.

Sequela

The patient does well and is able to be discharged from the hospital after a short stay. A week postoperatively, the patient returns with worsening pain and new feculent drainage from the incision.

What's the Working Diagnosis?

You are concerned about a superficial surgical site infection versus an enterocutaneous fistula. A CT fistulogram demonstrates fistulous connection from one of the surgical sites to the incision.

What's the Treatment Plan?

You admit the patient nil per os and start IV nutrition and antibiotics. You pouch the area of drainage to monitor output and protect the surrounding skin. You obtain baseline nutrition parameters.

Sequela

The patient improves on bowel rest and the fistula only drains 100 cc of succus a day. You slowly advance diet and monitor output. The output does not change. You are able to discharge the patient with the low-output fistula (<200 cc/24 h) with plans to reinitiate biologic therapy. You counsel the patient that biologic therapy may be able to facilitate spontaneous fistula closure or at least put her disease into remission prior to surgical fistula takedown.

The Scenario Changes

Instead of 100 cc, the fistula puts out 600 cc a day.

What's the Working Diagnosis?

This is a high-output fistula (>500 cc/24 h). The patient must remain nil per os on IV nutrition. You consider pharmacologic reduction of effluent with proton pump inhibitors, anti-motility agents, or antisecretory agents such as octreotide.

Case Scenario

A 23-year-old man presents to the emergency room with two days of right lower quadrant pain in addition to fevers, chills, nausea and vomiting, and focal tenderness on exam. His labwork is positive for leukocytosis with left shift.

What's the Working Diagnosis?

You are concerned about acute appendicitis (Table 4.1).

Table 4.1 Differential diagnosis for right lower quadrant abdominal pain

Gastroenteritis
Appendicitis
Inflammatory bowel disease
Gallstone ileus
Meckel's diverticulitis
Kidney stone/cystitis

What's Your Treatment Plan?

You admit the patient nil per os, start intravenous antibiotics, and obtain cross-sectional imaging. A CT scan reveals a dilated and inflamed appendix. You consent the patient for a laparoscopic appendectomy.

Operative Steps

Laparoscopic Appendectomy

1. Position the patient supine with left arm tucked and decompress the bladder and stomach.
2. Insufflate the abdomen and place three ports at the umbilicus, in the left lower quadrant, and in the suprapubic region.
3. Mobilize and identify the appendix, transect at the base, and divide the appendiceal mesentery.
4. Retrieve in a specimen bag and evaluate the remainder of the abdomen for alternative pathology if the appendix appears non-inflamed.

Sequela

The pathology report states the appendix contained a goblet cell adenocarcinoma, 1 cm in size near the midportion of the appendix.

What's the Treatment Plan?

You refer the patient for genetic testing given his young age, present his case at a multidisciplinary tumor board, and ultimately recommend oncologic right hemicolectomy to the patient (Table 4.2). You plan to prepare the patient to undergo surgery with an enhanced recovery after surgery protocol.

Table 4.2 Recommended treatment for incidental appendiceal tumors

Adenocarcinoma	Low-grade appendiceal mucinous neoplasm or T1 well-differentiated negative margins	Can consider observation after multidisciplinary tumor discussion
	All others	Right hemicolectomy
Carcinoid	<1 cm	Nothing further
	1–2 cm	Surveillance
	>2 cm	Appropriate staging and right hemicolectomy

Operative Steps

Laparoscopic Right Hemicolectomy (Fig. 4.1)

1. Mobilize the right colon in a medial to lateral fashion, taking care to protect the duodenum and performing high ligation of the ileocolic pedicle.
2. Transect the proximal transverse colon and the terminal ileum, taking care to identify and protect the ureter.
3. Mobilize the white line of Toldt and extract the specimen through an enlarged incision (midline, Pfannenstiel, etc.).
4. Perform an intracorporeal or extracorporeal stapled anastomosis.

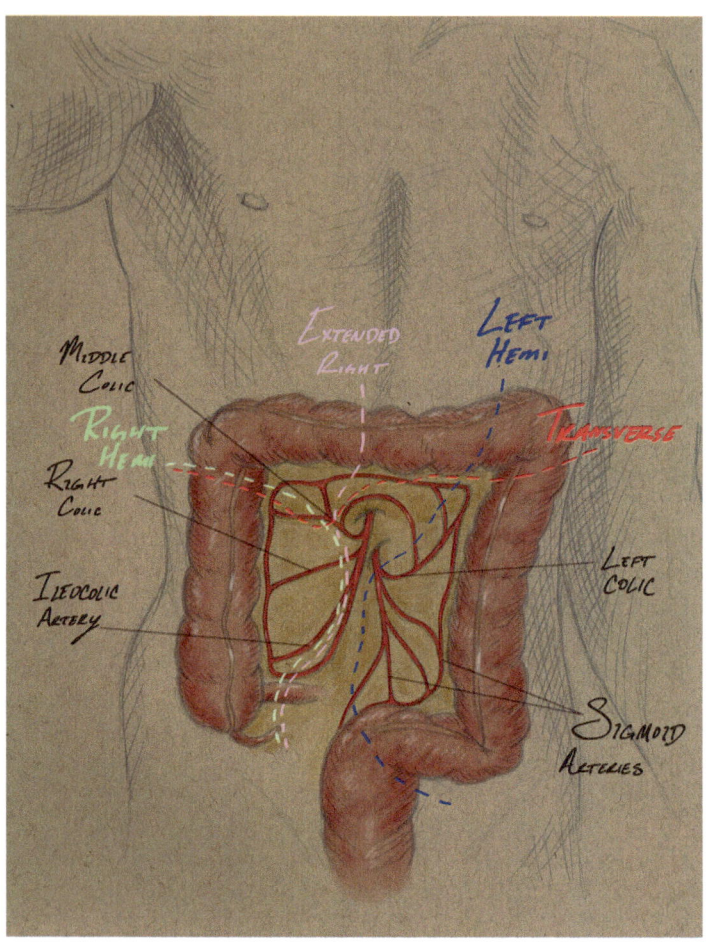

Fig. 4.1 Anatomic oncologic colon resections

Sequela

The night of surgery, you are called by the nurse who reports the patient is acutely tachycardic and hypotensive.

What's Your Next Step?

You promptly see and examine the patient and ensure there are at least two large bore IVs for access. You bolus a liter of crystalloid and send off a panel of labs. The patient is transiently responsive to the fluid bolus. His abdomen is distended and quite tender. Stat labs reveal a hemoglobin drop by three points.

What's the Treatment Plan?

You order emergency blood transfusion and plan to take the patient back for emergent exploration for presumed hemorrhage.

Case Scenario

A 45-year-old woman presents for her first screening colonoscopy. She is asymptomatic but concerned given her father had colon cancer at age 65. She has a long-standing history of constipation.

Operative Steps

Colonoscopy

1. Position the patient in left lateral decubitus.
2. Under monitored anesthesia care, perform an external visual and digital exam, followed by intubation of the anus with the scope.
3. Insert the scope until the cecum is reached, identifiable by the appendiceal orifice, the ileocecal valve, and the crow's foot landmark of the converging longitudinal bands.
4. Withdraw the scope using at minimum 6 min of duration, taking care to examine all mucosal surfaces.

Sequela

You identify a pedunculated polyp in the transverse colon and perform a snare polypectomy. You explain this finding to the patient upon recovery and the patient wishes to know when she needs another scope. You advise her that it is dependent on the findings on pathology, but likely a singular tubular adenoma would warrant a 7–10-year interval.

The Scenario Changes

You are unable to advance to the hepatic flexure.

What's Your Next Step?

You attempt to retract with a counterclockwise twist to undo any loops, ask an assistant to apply abdominal pressure, increase stiffness of the scope, or reposition the patient supine. Despite these maneuvers, you are unable to progress further.

Sequela

You opt to abort the procedure and send the patient for a virtual colonography.

The Scenario Changes

In the recovery room after an uneventful colonoscopy, the patient complains of severe abdominal pain. You assess the patient and are concerned for peritoneal signs.

What's the Working Diagnosis?

You are concerned about perforation and obtain a stat upright plain film. There is concern for free air. You consent the patient for emergent diagnostic laparoscopy, possible laparotomy. In the operating room, you find a large perforation in the sigmoid colon, greater than 50% of the circumference.

Operative Steps

Laparoscopic Left Colectomy

1. Position the patient supine in lithotomy with arms tucked; decompress the stomach and bladder.
2. Gain access and insufflate the abdomen.
3. Place three to four ports in the right abdomen; tilt the patient's left side up.
4. Perform medial to lateral or lateral to medial dissection, identifying and protecting the ureter.
5. Dissect and ligate the inferior mesenteric artery.
6. Free the colon from splenic flexure to sacral promontory and staple transect and extract the specimen (Table 4.3).
7. Perform stapled anastomosis and test for leak; consider leaving a pelvic drain.
8. Create a diverting loop ileostomy in specific circumstances such as high tension, tenuous blood supply, significant dissection, or high-risk comorbidities.

Table 4.3 Techniques to enable colon reach for a pelvic anastomosis

Divide the inferior mesenteric vein
Mobilize the splenic flexure
Divide the omental attachments to the transverse colon
Incise the colonic mesentery just medial to the middle colic vessels

Table 4.4 Alternative options for ureteral injury not amenable to simple repair

Ligate and reimplant directly into the bladder
Ligate and reimplant with psoas hitch and/or Boari flap to overcome distance
Ligate and obtain placement of percutaneous nephrostomy tube

During your operation, you notice an abrupt leakage of clear fluid along the inferior lateral dissection. You identify a partial ureteral injury at the pelvic brim (Table 4.4).

Operative Steps

Ureteral Repair (Fig. 4.2)

1. Debride back to healthy edges and spatulate the ends.
2. Pass a stent in the ureter across the injury.
3. Repair primarily over the stent with running absorbable monofilament.
4. Leave a catheter for bladder decompression.

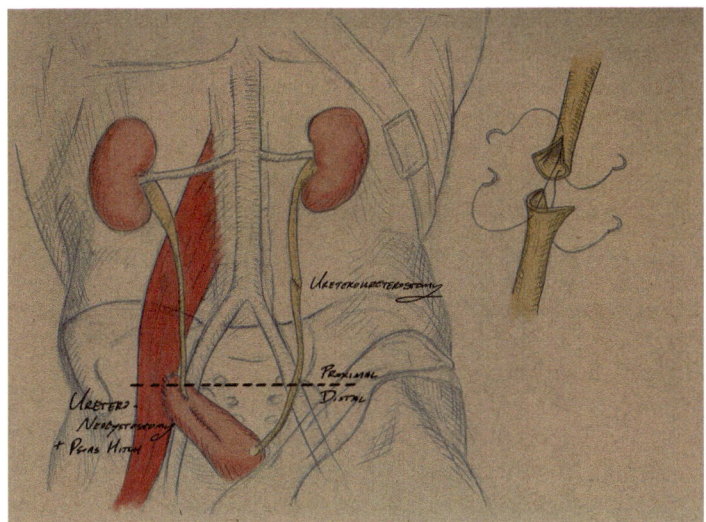

Fig. 4.2 Urinary tract injury repair

Sequela

You opted not to divert the patient due to having had a bowel prep for their colonoscopy and minimal contamination. On postoperative day five, the patient begins to have fevers and worsening abdominal pain. Labwork reveals a leukocytosis. You obtain cross-sectional imaging which reveals a fluid and gas collection abutting the stapled anastomosis. In addition, there are distant dots of free air.

What's the Working Diagnosis?

You are concerned for an anastomotic leak leading to the deep organ space infection.

What's the Treatment Plan?

You counsel the patient on the radiographic findings and consent the patient for washout and diversion with a loop ileostomy. The patient wishes to know if the ostomy is permanent.

You advise that pending recovery and healing, ileostomy reversal could be undertaken in 3–6 months.

Operative Steps

Brooke Loop Ileostomy

1. Select a loop of ileum proximal to the ileocecal valve with enough reach to protrude through the abdomen without undue tension.
2. Excise a circular column of skin and soft tissue overlying the rectus muscle.
3. Create a cruciate incision in the fascia, split the rectus muscle, and incise the posterior fascial sheath.
4. Bring out the ileum and close any other abdominal incisions.
5. Create an enterotomy.
6. Place interrupted sutures with a mucosal bite, a seromuscular bite, and then a skin bite to create a rosebud effect of the afferent os (Fig. 4.3).

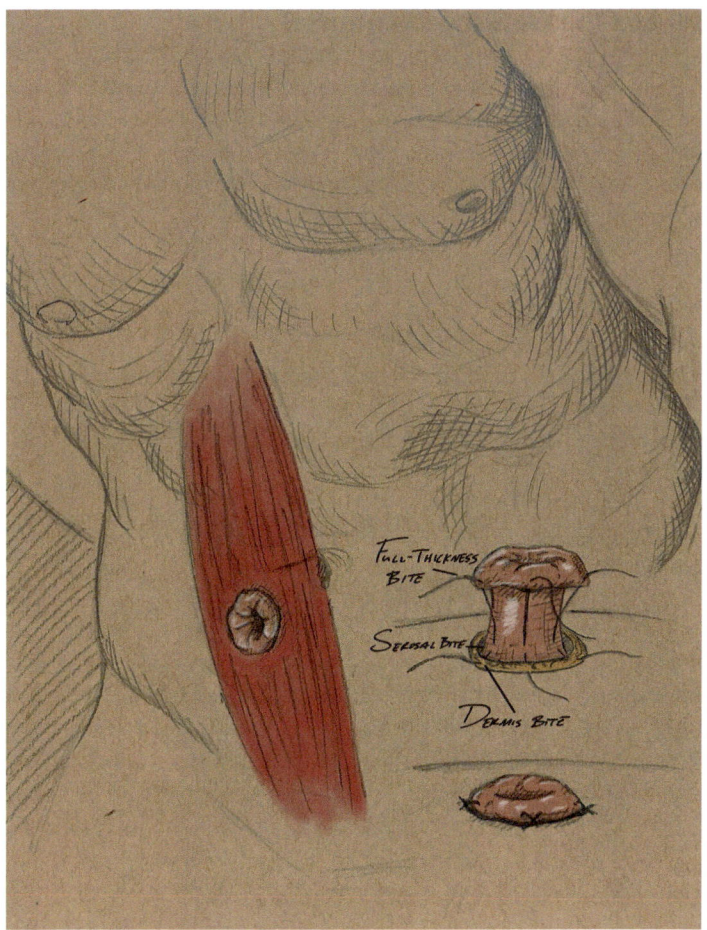

Fig. 4.3 Maturing an ileostomy in the Brooke fashion

Case Scenario

A 36-year-old transgender woman comes to you with complaints of three days of pain and swelling near their anus. She has noticed some chills. She feels the swelling has been increasing.

What's the Working Diagnosis?

You are concerned about possible perianal abscess versus a thrombosed external hemorrhoid. You examine the patient and conclude that it is an abscess. You perform an incision and drainage in the office. The patient improves, but returns three months later with a recurrent abscess at the same location.

What's Your Next Step?

You are concerned about a fistula leading to recurrent abscesses. You consent the patient for exam under anesthesia with possibility of fistulotomy versus seton placement if a fistula-in-ano is identified.

Sequela

You find that the fistula is transsphincteric and involves greater than a third of the sphincter muscle, prompting placement of a seton. The patient improves but wants to know when the seton can be removed. You counsel the patient on waiting 8–12 weeks prior to secondary intervention (Table 4.5).

Table 4.5 Interventions for complex anorectal fistula

Perform ligation of the intersphincteric fistula tract for transsphincteric fistula
Perform endorectal advancement flap
Place fistula plug or fibrin glue

The Scenario Changes

The patient instead reports acute sharp pain with bowel movements, ever since one particular hard stool. On exam, you identify a posterior midline fissure.

What's the Treatment Plan?

You advise the patient on conservative measures including sitz baths, stool softeners, adequate hydration, and fiber intake and prescribe a trial of diltiazem cream.

The patient follows your recommendations to the letter but ultimately still complains of symptoms. You consent the patient for lateral internal sphincterotomy.

Operative Steps

Lateral Internal Sphincterotomy

1. Position the patient prone jackknife under general anesthesia.
2. Examine the anus and anal canal to confirm diagnosis of fissure without any other anomaly.
3. Incise the mucosa overlying the intersphincteric groove on the right lateral side of the anal canal.
4. Using a blunt dissector, open the intersphincteric space and elevate a segment of internal sphincter to divide.
5. Divide the sphincter muscle, taking care not to extend beyond the dentate line.
6. Ensure hemostasis and either suture close or leave the incision open.

The Scenario Changes

Instead of a fissure, you identify swollen prolapsed internal hemorrhoids. They reduce on manual pressure but spontaneously prolapse easily. The patient has already tried hydrocortisone cream and other nonoperative interventions. The patient would like to proceed with surgical hemorrhoidectomy.

Operative Steps

Hemorrhoidectomy

1. Position the patient in either prone jackknife or high lithotomy under general anesthesia.
2. Examine the anus and anal canal to confirm the diagnosis without any other anomaly present.
3. Grasping the largest hemorrhoid first, place a suture ligature at the feeding vessel at the apex of the hemorrhoid.
4. Transect the hemorrhoid with cautery or sharply, taking care not to incorporate the underlying sphincter muscle.
5. Ensure hemostasis and either suture close or leave open the wound.

Sequela

On final pathology, the specimen contained a 3 cm squamous cell cancer on the hemorrhoid, negative margins. You counsel the patient on the finding and reexamine the groins, finding no adenopathy. You obtain staging imaging and present the case at a multidisciplinary tumor board. The recommendation is to proceed with Nigro protocol, which consists of 45 Gy radiation therapy plus mitomycin C and 5-fluorouracil chemotherapies.

The patient undergoes the recommended treatment but develops recurrent disease two years later.

What's the Treatment Plan?

For recurrent or residual disease after Nigro protocol, you counsel the patient on salvage abdominoperineal resection. You consider involvement of plastic surgery for potential flap closure of the perineum.

Operative Steps

Abdominoperineal Resection

1. Position the patient in supine lithotomy under general anesthesia.
2. Access the abdominal cavity and confirm no intraperitoneal disease.
3. Perform the pelvic dissection, entering the presacral space posterior to the rectum and dissecting down to the levator ani.
4. Complete the total mesorectal dissection laterally and anteriorly, taking care to preserve the pelvic nerves, ureters, and presacral veins.
5. Divide the proximal mesentery, preserving the inferior mesenteric artery, and transect the sigmoid colon with a stapler.
6. Create and bring up the end colostomy.
7. Proceed to the perineal portion, suture close the anus, and incise the perianal verge in an extrasphincteric fashion.
8. Connect the perineal and abdominal dissection and remove the specimen.
9. Suture close the perineum in layers and consider flap coverage and drain placement.
10. Mature the end colostomy after closing the abdomen.

Additional Reading

1. Bleier JIS, Beck DE, Wexner SD, Rafferty JF, Gordon PH, Hatch Q, et al. Gordon and Nivatvongs' principles and practice of surgery for the colon, Rectum, and Anus. Stuttgart: Georg Thieme Verlag; 2019.
2. Burks FN, Santucci RA. Management of iatrogenic ureteral injury. Ther Adv Urol. 2014;6(3):115–24. https://doi.org/10.1177/1756287214526767. PMID: 24883109; PMCID: PMC4003841.
3. Haycock A, Cohen J, Saunders B, Cotton PB, Williams CB. Cotton and Williams' practical gastrointestinal endoscopy: the fundamentals. Chichester: Wiley; 2014.
4. National Comprehensive Cancer Network. Colon cancer. In: NCCN clinical practice guidelines in oncology; 2024. https://www.nccn.org/professionals/physician_gls/pdf/colon.pdf. Accessed 30 Dec 2024.
5. National Comprehensive Cancer Network. Squamous cell skin cancer. In: NCCN clinical practice guidelines in oncology. 2024. https://www.nccn.org/professionals/physician_gls/pdf/squamous.pdf. Accessed 30 Dec 2024.

Abdominal Cavity and Hernia

5

Case Scenario

A 53-year-old man presents to your office in referral from nephrology. He has stage V chronic kidney disease and is anticipated to start dialysis imminently. He has discussed the options for dialysis and wishes to proceed with peritoneal dialysis. He has never had abdominal surgery.

What's Your Next Step?

After confirming peritoneal dialysis candidacy (Table 5.1), you consent the patient for placement of a peritoneal dialysis catheter.

© The Author(s), under exclusive license to Springer Nature Switzerland AG 2025
S. Hao et al., *General Surgery Boards Case-Based Review*, https://doi.org/10.1007/978-3-031-85631-0_5

Table 5.1 Contraindications to peritoneal dialysis

Active abdominal infection
Ischemic bowel
Active inflammatory bowel disease
Inability to care for peritoneal catheter (psychiatric, physical, or
intellectual limitations)
Pregnancy
Loss of peritoneal membrane or membrane defects (such as an ostomy)
Extensive intra-abdominal scarring
Liver disease with ascites

Operative Steps

Placement of Peritoneal Dialysis Catheter

1. With the patient supine under general anesthesia, access the abdominal cavity at the umbilicus.
2. Feed in the catheter on the stylet aiming for the pelvis.
3. Obtain a plain film to confirm pelvic location of the distal tip; then remove the stylet.
4. Secure the deep cuff to the fascia.
5. Tunnel the midportion of the catheter under the skin and subcutaneous tissue to a selected exit site, leaving the superficial cuff within the tunnel.
6. Connect the midportion and the peritoneal portion and suture close any incisions.
7. Connect the exit site to a dialysate bag and test for both instillation by gravity and adequate drainage by gravity.
8. Obtain a plain film to confirm final location of the spiraled catheter tip.

Sequela

The patient initiates peritoneal dialysis but encounters difficulty with fully draining after about a month of dialysis.

What's the Working Diagnosis?

The patient is having catheter malfunction. This may be due to constipation, catheter malposition or kink, catheter fibrin clog, intra-abdominal adhesions, or omental wrapping. The nephrologist obtained a plain film confirming correct location of the catheter tip and has attempted several doses of alteplase per catheter with no success.

What's the Treatment Plan?

You consent the patient for diagnostic laparoscopy to attempt to diagnose and treat the cause of catheter malfunction, with the possibility of replacing the catheter.

In the operating room, you identify and lyse adhesions and test the catheter instillation and drainage with successful results. The patient returns three days later with severe abdominal pain and reports the effluent has been rather cloudy.

What's the Working Diagnosis?

You are concerned about catheter-associated peritonitis. You admit the patient and start broad-spectrum intraperitoneal antibiotics and send the effluent for culture.

Case Scenario

A 76-year-old woman presents to your office to discuss options for her large ventral hernia. She has previously undergone bariatric surgery which was complicated by an internal hernia requiring emergent laparotomy and bowel resection. This left her with the current hernia. She has regained some weight and her current body mass index (BMI) is 32. She has never had any surgical attempts to repair the hernia. She does have a history of coronary artery disease with prior remote myocardial infarction on daily aspirin, hypertension, diabetes mellitus with hemoglobin A1c of 7%, and mild chronic obstructive pulmonary disease not on oxygen. She quit smoking a year ago. She performs her own independent activities of daily living including weekly yoga.

What's the Next Step?

For an elective surgery, you advise on the need to determine her cardiopulmonary risk for surgery and optimize her status. You counsel her on reduced hernia recurrence with a BMI < 30 if she is able to achieve it prior to proceeding.

You obtain a 12-lead EKG based on her current elevated cardiac risk. The EKG appears unchanged from baseline. The patient is able to achieve some weight loss with lifestyle changes and is eager to proceed.

Operative Steps

Ventral Hernia Repair

1. Position the patient supine under general anesthesia.
2. Incise the skin and dissect down to the hernia sac, taking care not to injure underlying hernia contents such as bowel.
3. Remove the hernia sac and identify healthy fascial edges.
4. Measure the defect distance and test for tension if the fascial edges are reapproximated.
5. Place a synthetic mesh large enough to cover a margin beyond the fascial defect in the peritoneal or preperitoneal space.
6. Primarily close the fascia with running monofilament nonabsorbable suture.
7. Close the subcutaneous space and skin with consideration for drain placement.

The Scenario Changes

Suppose, intraoperatively, the fascial edges do not come together and the defect is 15 cm wide. Preoperatively, you would have discussed the possibility of needing component separation in order to bridge the defect.

Operative Steps

Abdominal Component Separation

1. Elevate subcutaneous flaps taking care to preserve perforators.
2. For an anterior approach, incise the external oblique fascia 2 cm lateral from the rectus sheath from costal to inguinal borders (Fig. 5.1).
3. For a posterior approach, incise the posterior rectus sheath just medial to the linea semilunaris, avoiding the neurovascular supply to the rectus.
4. Place mesh either in an inlay fashion within the muscle layers for anterior reinforcement or in a retrorectus fashion for posterior reinforcement.
5. Close the mobilized fascial edges.
6. Close skin and subcutaneous tissue over drains.

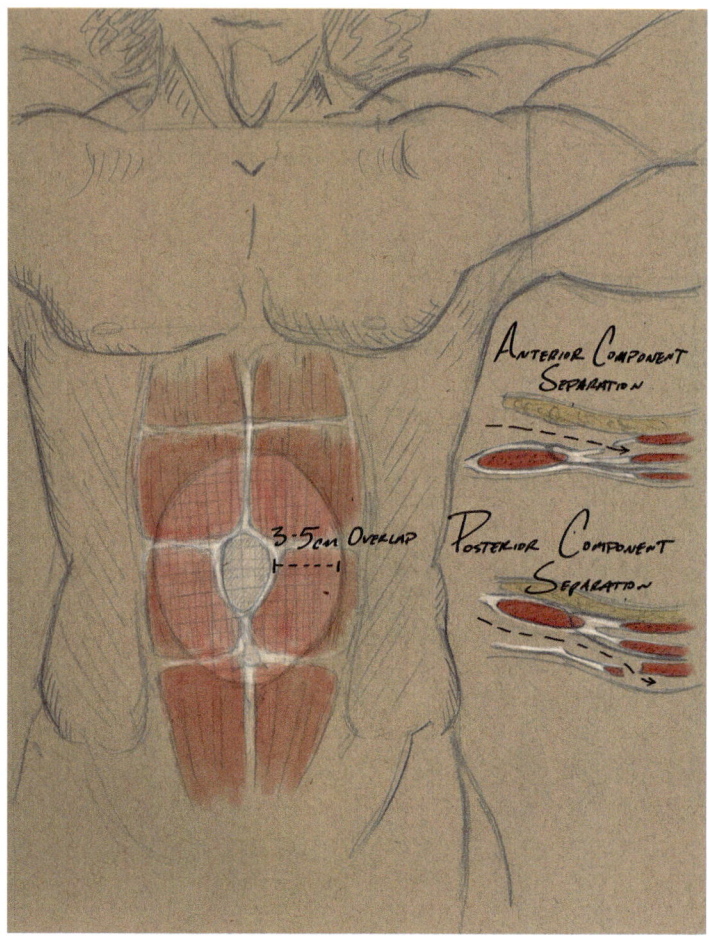

Fig. 5.1 Ventral hernia repair with component separation diagrams

Sequela

For the patient who underwent repair without component separation, she returns 2 weeks later with erythema and tenderness at her incision. You palpate some fluctuance.

What's the Working Diagnosis?

You are concerned about a surgical site infection. You incise a portion of the incision and release purulent fluid. You gently probe the cavity and are able to palpate a fascial defect and the mesh itself. You are now concerned about mesh infection.

What's the Treatment Plan?

You discuss the need to control the infection with adequate drainage, debridement to healthy tissue, and wound management techniques such as vacuum dressings. You counsel on the possibility of needing to explant infected mesh and bridge with temporary absorbable mesh with the expectation of future repeat attempt at definitive hernia repair.

Case Scenario

A 41-year-old man who works in construction presents to the emergency room with acute groin pain. He believes he has had a chronic groin hernia which is now "stuck." He is having nausea and vomiting.

What's the Working Diagnosis?

You are concerned about an incarcerated inguinal or femoral hernia leading to bowel obstruction. The differential for groin pain includes gonadal torsion, groin abscess, hydrocele, or an inflamed and enlarged lymph node.

On exam, you identify a left inguinal hernia which is swollen, erythematous, and tender. It is not reducible (Table 5.2). The patient's bloodwork reveals a leukocytosis. The patient's abdomen is also distended.

Table 5.2 Techniques for bedside groin hernia reduction

Provide analgesia or conscious sedation
Tilt the bed to gain the assistance of gravity
Apply gentle steady pressure
Align or guide the hernia contents along the anatomical opening, which
may require pulling or lengthening the hernia sac

What's the Treatment Plan?

You are now concerned for strangulation. You opt not to attempt to reduce the hernia given the concern for strangulation and the need to both evaluate the bowel and proceed to the operating room in a timely fashion. You discuss with the patient the need to proceed to urgent exploration to reduce and repair the hernia, with the possibility of bowel resection. You place a nasogastric tube for decompression prior to proceeding.

Operative Steps

Open Inguinal Hernia Repair (Bassini or Lichtenstein)

1. With the patient supine under general or spinal anesthesia, make an oblique incision 2 fingerbreadths above an imaginary line drawn from anterior superior iliac spine to pubis.
2. Dissect down to the external oblique fascia, ligating the superficial epigastric artery if needed.
3. Incise the external oblique fascia sharply along its fibers, taking care not to injure the underlying ilioinguinal nerve.
4. Encircle the hernia and canal contents and separate the cord structures from hernia sac (Fig. 5.2).
5. Isolate the cord structures with a silastic drain or vessel loop.
6. Open the hernia sac and inspect the bowel.
7. Resect any frankly necrotic bowel; otherwise reduce the contents into the peritoneal cavity.
8. Ligate and resect the hernia sac at the neck.

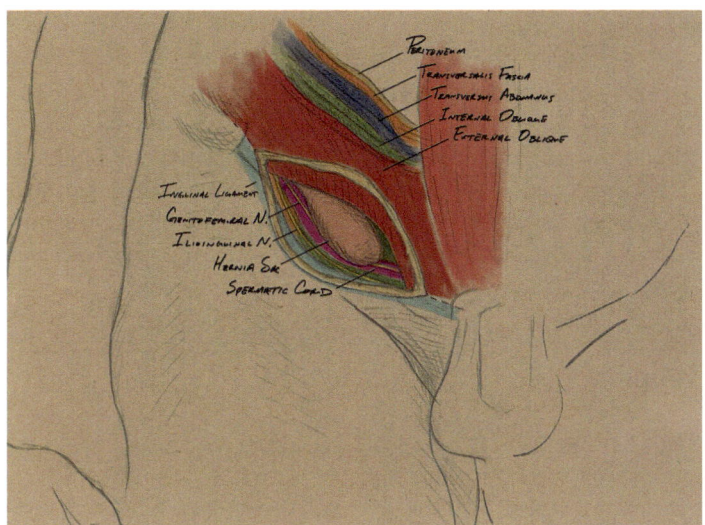

Fig. 5.2 Anatomy of inguinal hernia repair

9. Close the floor of the inguinal canal by suturing the conjoint tendon to the inguinal ligament with monofilament nonabsorbable running suture (Bassini), or secure prosthetic mesh to the pubic tubercle, conjoint tendon, and inguinal ligament (Lichtenstein) with monofilament nonabsorbable suture.
10. Close the external oblique fascia and skin and return the testes to anatomical position if needed.
11. Explore the abdomen open or laparoscopically if the reduced bowel needs to be reexamined or an anastomosis needs to be performed.

The Scenario Changes

As you explore the inguinal hernia, you identify that the hernia is in fact a femoral hernia.

Operative Steps

Open Femoral Hernia Repair (McVay)

1. Following reduction and resection of the hernia sac, suture the conjoint tendon to the pectineal ligament at the pubic bone (Cooper's ligament) with nonabsorbable monofilament suture.
2. Recreate the anatomic internal ring by suturing the transversalis fascia to the iliopubic tract.

Sequela

Years later, the patient returns to your office with recurrence in the left- as well as a right-sided inguinal hernia. He wants to know his options for repair. You discuss the possibilities of repeat open repair, an intra-abdominal approach with peritoneal mesh placement, or a preperitoneal approach with mesh placement. The latter approaches would allow bilateral repair at the same time.

Case Scenario

A 68-year-old woman with severe alcoholic cirrhosis with ascites presents to your office for evaluation of an umbilical hernia. She has had an umbilical hernia for many years, but lately she feels the hernia has been increasing in size. On exam, the umbilical hernia has a 5 cm defect and the overlying skin is quite thin. The patient's abdomen is protuberant and has a fluid wave. There are stigmata of liver disease including recanalized umbilical veins. You determine that she has Childs-Pugh class C liver disease.

What's the Treatment Plan?

You counsel the patient on the high perioperative risk associated with elective repair as well as the morbidity of urgent repair should hernia complications arise. You ensure the patient sees hepatology to optimize ascites and disease control (Table 5.3).

Table 5.3 Medical management of cirrhosis with ascites

Low sodium diet
Diuretics
Paracentesis
Beta-blockade
Resolution of underlying cause (hepatitis, alcohol consumption, etc.)
Evaluation for transjugular intrahepatic portosystemic shunt (TIPS)
candidacy if significant portal hypertension
Evaluation for transplant candidacy

Sequela

You are called to see the patient in the emergency room. The patient was sent directly from the office of the hepatologist after the physician noted spontaneous rupture. This was the patient's first visit to hepatology and no new therapy has been initiated. On exam, there is clear fluid leaking from a punctate skin defect overlying the hernia.

What's Your Next Step?

You admit the patient, initiate prophylactic antibiotics, and initiate steps to obtain ascites control. You apply a sterile dressing. The patient undergoes paracentesis with albumin replacement therapy and is started on diuretics. The fluid leak persists and you consent the patient for herniorrhaphy.

Operative Steps

Open Umbilical Hernia Repair

1. Make a longitudinal incision over the hernia defect.
2. Reduce any hernia contents and resect the hernia sac.
3. Elevate subcutaneous flaps if necessary to allow fascial closure.

4. Suture the fascial edges together with monofilament nonabsorbable running suture.
5. Resect any devitalized skin.
6. Close skin and subcutaneous tissue in layers.

Sequela

The patient is able to achieve optimal management of her disease and ascites including TIPS procedure prior to discharge from the hospital. Although the hernia does recur, she completes candidacy evaluation and undergoes liver transplantation with definitive hernia repair at the time.

Additional Reading

1. Bulyk I, Shkarban V, Vasyliuk S, Osadets V, Bitska I, Dmytruk O. The history of inguinal hernia surgery. Rozhl Chir. 2023;102(4):149–53. https://doi.org/10.33699/PIS.2023.102.4.149-153.   English.   PMID: 37344194.
2. Karkar A, Wilkie M. Peritoneal dialysis in the modern era. Perit Dial Int. 2023;43(4):301–14. https://doi.org/10.1177/08968608221114211. Epub 2022 Aug 3. PMID: 35923087.
3. Liang MK, Holihan JL, Itani K, Alawadi ZM, Gonzalez JR, Askenasy EP, Ballecer C, Chong HS, Goldblatt MI, Greenberg JA, Harvin JA, Keith JN, Martindale RG, Orenstein S, Richmond B, Roth JS, Szotek P, Towfigh S, Tsuda S, Vaziri K, Berger DH. Ventral hernia management: expert consensus guided by systematic review. Ann Surg. 2017;265(1):80–9. https://doi.org/10.1097/SLA.0000000000001701. PMID: 28009730
4. Pawlak M, East B, de Beaux AC. Algorithm for management of an incarcerated inguinal hernia in the emergency settings with manual reduction. Taxis, the technique and its safety. Hernia. 2021;25(5):1253–8. https://doi.org/10.1007/s10029-021-02429-1. Epub 2021 May 25. PMID: 34036484; PMCID: PMC8147903. PMID: 35507128.
5. Bronswijk M, Jaekers J, Vanella G, Struyve M, Miserez M, van der Merwe S. Umbilical hernia repair in patients with cirrhosis: who, when and how to treat. Hernia. 2022;26(6):1447–57. https://doi.org/10.1007/s10029-022-02617-7. Epub 2022 May 4.
6. Sanchez VM, Abi-Haidar YE, Itani KM. Mesh infection in ventral incisional hernia repair: incidence, contributing factors, and treatment. Surg Infect. 2011;12(3):205–10. https://doi.org/10.1089/sur.2011.033. Epub 2011 Jul 18. PMID: 21767146.

Skin/Soft Tissue

6

Case Scenario

An 88-year-old man presents for evaluation of an abnormal lesion on his lower back. He cannot see it but his partner noted that the lesion seems to have grown. He has also noted intermittent blood spotting on his shirt. He often worked in the sun during his lifetime with his back exposed without sunscreen use. He has no other comorbidities and remains active. He is thin. On exam, you note a 3 cm irregularly shaped black and brown flat lesion with some areas of ulceration. There is no palpable adenopathy.

What's the Working Diagnosis?

You are concerned about a melanoma (Table 6.1). You obtain a punch biopsy.

The punch biopsy reveals a 1-mm-thick melanoma with ulcerations.

Table 6.1 Differential diagnoses of skin lesions

Melanoma
Basal cell carcinoma
Squamous cell precursor lesions or carcinoma
Benign nevus or birthmarks
Paget's disease
Skin infections such as folliculitis or tinea
Inflammatory lesions such as erythema multiforme or eczema

What's the Treatment Plan?

You present the case at a multidisciplinary tumor board. Based on the recommendations, you discuss wide local excision with 1–2 cm margins and sentinel lymph node biopsy. You counsel the patient on the potential need for flap or graft closure should the defect not be amenable to primary closure. The patient agrees to proceed.

Prior to the procedure, you inject radionuclide into the dermal tissue in four quadrants around the lesion. The patient goes to nuclear imaging and undergoes nuclear scintigraphy. The lesion appears to drain into the right groin.

Operative Steps

Inguinal Sentinel Lymph Node Biopsy for Melanoma

1. Prior to making the wide local excision incision, inject isosulfan blue dye into the dermal tissue in four quadrants around the lesion.
2. Make a vertical incision along the medial thigh spanning the inferior edge of the inguinal ligament to the apex of the femoral triangle.
3. Using a gamma probe, identify and excise any nodes that have radioactive counts greater than ten times the background count, even if they are not blue.

4. Identify and excise any nodes that are visibly blue, even if not radioactive.
5. Inspect and excise any palpably pathologic nodes even if neither blue nor radioactive.
6. Ensure hemostasis and close in layers.

Wide Local Excision for Melanoma

1. Mark an elliptical resection that is at least 1–2 cm away from all borders of the visible lesion, oriented along Langer lines.
2. Carry the incision down to the level of the fascia, and then excise the specimen off of the fascia.
3. Orient the specimen cranially/caudally and medially/laterally with sutures or clips.
4. Close the incision in layers if able to approximate without tension.

You determine that due to the patient's lack of redundant tissue, the edges do not reapproximate. A rotational or regional flap is not possible either. You opt to harvest a split thickness graft.

The Scenario Changes

You have instead performed the procedure on a melanoma of the elbow with the same difficulty of closing the incision. You opt to perform a full thickness skin graft.

Operative Steps

Full Thickness Skin Graft

1. Create a template of the defect and outline the donor site (Table 6.2) based on the template.
2. Harvest the donor site down to the level of adipose with minimal use of cautery.

Table 6.2 Possible donor sites for full thickness skin grafts

Back
Abdominal wall
Supraclavicular
Preauricular
Postauricular
Forehead
Inner upper arm

3. Ensure hemostasis and perform primary closure or split thickness grafting of the donor site.
4. Defat the graft and secure to recipient bed with sutures and pressure bolster.
5. Leave in place for 1 week.

Sequela

One of the four sentinel nodes excised is positive for micrometastasis. You re-present the patient at the multidisciplinary tumor board. Per the Multicenter Selective Lymphadenectomy Trial II (MSLT-2), there is no survival benefit to pursuing inguinal node dissection although there is a benefit for local disease control. The patient wishes to avoid nodal dissection. Based on the recommendations, you obtain staging imaging and *BRAF* mutation testing. Imaging does not reveal any metastatic disease.

You refer the patient to oncology for consideration of checkpoint inhibitor adjuvant therapy such as nivolumab or pembrolizumab, or dabrafenib if BRAF V600 mutation positive. You plan to surveil the patient with complete skin and nodal exam every six months for two years, and then annually thereafter, as well as nodal basin ultrasound every six months for two years.

Case Scenario

A 40-year-old woman presents to your office for evaluation of a thigh mass. She is unsure of how long she has had it but feels it has become more noticeable in the past year. It is palpated to about 6 cm in diameter and is nontender, mobile, soft, and somewhat lobulated. She has no other symptoms or findings on exam. Her routine bloodwork obtained recently by her primary care provider is unremarkable.

What's the Working Diagnosis?

You suspect this may be a benign lipoma, although soft tissue lesions can be sarcomatous, infectious, or of neurologic origin such as a ganglion cyst or neuroma. You obtain an ultrasound to further characterize the lesion. On ultrasound, there are microcalcifications and it is unclear if the lesion has a separate plane from the underlying muscle fascia.

What's Your Next Step?

You obtain a core biopsy. The pathology indicates benign adipose tissue. A second core biopsy is equally uninformative. The patient consents to proceeding with incisional versus excisional biopsy.

Operative Steps

Incisional Extremity Soft Tissue Mass Biopsy

1. Incise longitudinally directly overlying the mass.
2. Dissect down to the mass.
3. Sharply transect a portion for pathology.
4. Obtain hemostasis and close in layers.

Excisional Extremity Soft Tissue Mass Biopsy

1. Make an elliptical incision overlying the mass and incorporating any prior core biopsy entry points on the skin.
2. Carry the incision down to the mass.
3. Dissect out the mass taking care not to violate a capsule if present.
4. If adhered or involving the underlying fascia, incorporate the fascia into the specimen.
5. Orient the specimen with sutures or clips.
6. Obtain hemostasis and close in layers, with consideration for drain placement in a large cavity.

Sequela

The pathology returns well-differentiated liposarcoma with negative margins. However the patient fails to show up for her postoperative check and planned drain removal. A week later, you arc called to the emergency room, where you find the patient has presented with significant pain and swelling of her operative extremity. There is crepitus and bullae. Erythema tracks up the lower back and across the groin. The pain is febrile, hypotensive, tachycardic, and somewhat confused. The drain was reportedly dislodged at some point and no longer present.

What's the Working Diagnosis?

You are concerned that a surgical site infection has developed with signs that it has become a necrotizing soft tissue or myofascial infection.

What's Your Next Step?

You initiate fluid resuscitation and broad-spectrum antibiotics and take the patient for wide debridement in order to obtain source control.

Operative Steps

Debridement of Necrotizing Infections

1. Position and drape the involved location and all possible areas of spread.
2. Excise overlying devitalized skin.
3. Remove all necrotic tissue and drain areas of pus.
4. Assess the depth of involvement (dermis, fascia, muscle, etc.).
5. Debride back to healthy bleeding tissue edges.
6. Ensure hemostasis and place temporary wet to dry gauze dressings with plans to return in 24 h for a second look.

Sequela

The patient is stabilized in the ICU and no further devitalized tissue is found at the second look. You opt to place a vacuum dressing to promote rapid tissue healing once the wound bed is felt to be clean.

Case Scenario

A 19-year-old obese man presents to your office for recurrent buttock abscesses. He reports they occur in the cleft between his gluteal cheeks. He has undergone several incision and drainage procedures in the emergency room. On exam you find extremely hairy skin in the natal cleft with prior scarring and pits. There is no fluctuance or cellulitis.

What's the Working Diagnosis?

Although hidradenitis may present with recurrent infections and scarred tissue with chronic sinuses, this occurs in skin with sweat glands. His symptoms specifically in the natal cleft are more consistent with pilonidal disease.

What's the Treatment Plan?

You advise the patient on conservative measures such as regular shaving or depilation or permanent laser hair removal, maintaining regular hygiene, and losing weight which may help. Infections would be treated with incision and drainage, and cellulitis would be treated with antibiotics. Persistent sinuses can be treated surgically with unroofing or curetting of the tracts, or complete excision with primary or flap closure (Fig. 6.1).

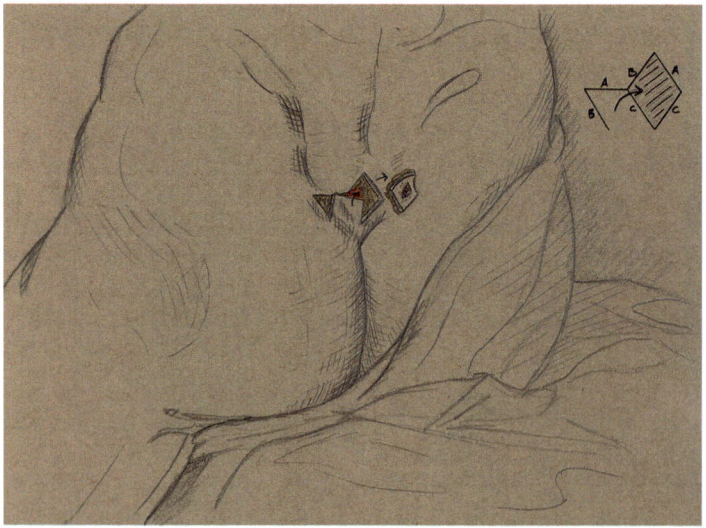

Fig. 6.1 Rotational rhomboid Limberg flap for pilonidal disease

Additional Reading

1. Bello DM, Faries MB. The landmark series: MSLT-1, MSLT-2 and DeCOG (Management of Lymph Nodes). Ann Surg Oncol. 2020;27(1):15–21. https://doi.org/10.1245/s10434-019-07830-w. Epub 2019 Sep 18. PMID: 31535299.
2. Bhama AR, Davis BR. Pilonidal disease and hidradenitis Suppurativa. In: ASCRS Textbook of Colon and Rectal Surgery. Springer; 2022. https://www.ascrsu.com/ascrs/view/ASCRS-Textbook-of-Colon-and-Rectal-Surgery/2285008/all/Pilonidal_Disease_and_Hidradenitis_Suppurativa. Accessed 30 Dec 2024.
3. McDermott J, Kao LS, Keeley JA, Grigorian A, Neville A, de Virgilio C. Necrotizing soft tissue infections: a review. JAMA Surg. 2024;159(11):1308–15. https://doi.org/10.1001/jamasurg.2024.3365. PMID: 39259555.
4. National Comprehensive Cancer Network. Melanoma: cutaneous. In: NCCN clinical practice guidelines in oncology; 2024. https://www.nccn.org/professionals/physician_gls/pdf/cutaneous_melanoma.pdf. Accessed 30 Dec 2024.
5. National Comprehensive Cancer Network. Soft tissue sarcoma. In: NCCN clinical practice guidelines in oncology; 2024. https://www.nccn.org/professionals/physician_gls/pdf/sarcoma.pdf. Accessed 30 Dec 2024.

Breast

7

Case Scenario

A 52-year-old woman presents to your office for evaluation of a lump she found in her left breast. She has had prior negative mammograms but missed several in a row due to the pandemic impacting her employment and insurance coverage. She has not noted any nipple discharge, any tenderness or erythema related to the lump, or skin changes. She has not experienced any breast trauma. On exam, there is subtle skin retraction at the palpable 2 cm lump in the upper outer quadrant, and the lump itself is hard and immobile. You do not palpate any adenopathy.

What's the Working Diagnosis?

You are concerned about a possible breast malignancy (Table 7.1).

You send the patient for bilateral diagnostic mammography and ultrasound of the axilla with a request to biopsy a lesion if found. On mammography, there is a 2 cm lesion reported as Breast Imaging Reporting & Data System (BI-RADS) category 4 (Table 7.2). The radiologist performs a core biopsy. The axillary ultrasound is negative.

The biopsy reveals ductal adenocarcinoma, ER and PR positive, HER2 negative.

Table 7.1 Differential breast mass pathology

Cyst
Galactocele
Male gynecomastia
Fibroadenoma
Fat necrosis
Malignancy

Table 7.2 BI-RADS categories, interpretation, and next step

BI-RADS 0	Incomplete	Obtain additional workup
BI-RADS 1	Normal imaging	Normal surveillance
BI-RADS 2	Benign finding	Normal surveillance
BI-RADS 3	Probably benign finding	Short-term surveillance versus biopsy
BI-RADS 4	Probably malignant finding	Obtain biopsy
BI-RADS 5	Malignant finding	Obtain biopsy
BI-RADS 6	Known breast malignancy	Proceed with planned treatment

What's the Treatment Plan?

You present the patient at a multidisciplinary tumor board. Based on their recommendations, you counsel the patient on the possibilities of lumpectomy with sentinel node biopsy in a breast conservation approach, versus a mastectomy with sentinel node biopsy. If mastectomy is pursued, you counsel the patient on speaking with a plastic surgeon regarding reconstruction if desired. The patient opts for a breast conservation approach.

Operative Steps

Axillary Sentinel Lymph Node Biopsy for Breast Cancer

1. Prior to the procedure, inject both isosulfan blue dye and radionuclide into the dermis in four quadrants around the nipple areola complex.
2. Make a transverse incision in the axilla, carry the incision down, and incise the clavipectoral fascia.
3. Using a gamma probe, identify and excise any nodes with a radioactive count greater than ten times the background count, even if not blue.
4. Inspect and excise any blue nodes even if not radioactive.
5. Inspect and excise any palpably pathologic nodes even if neither blue nor radioactive.
6. Obtain hemostasis and close in layers.

Lumpectomy or Partial Mastectomy

1. Make a curvilinear or radial incision overlying the mass.
2. Excise a globe of breast tissue encompassing the palpable mass.
3. Ensure hemostasis, place clips at the surgical margins, and close the incision.

Sequela

The pathology reveals a very close 1 mm deep margin and one lymph node involved with micrometastasis. You counsel the patient that despite the closeness, this still represents a negative oncologic margin (no tumor on ink). Based on the American College of Surgeons Oncology Group Z0011 (ACOSOG Z-11) trial, there was no survival benefit to pursuing complete axillary dissection with tumor involving one lymph node. The patient opts to avoid axillary dissection and complete adjuvant radiation. After re-presenting the case at the multidisciplinary tumor board, you refer the patient to oncology to initiate hormone therapy given the tumor receptor status.

Case Scenario

A 49-year-old obese male presents to your office with questions. He believes his family member tested positive for a breast cancer gene (BRCA) mutation and wonders about his breast cancer risk. He has been gaining weight recently without particular change to his diet and is fearful that his enlarging chest tissue may be underlying cancer. On exam, you note bilateral breast tissue without underlying palpable mass, no nipple or skin changes, and negative lymph node exam.

What's the Working Diagnosis?

Male breast enlargement may be gynecomastia, especially if bilateral and occurring in the setting of weight gain and other signs of hormonal imbalance. However, both BRCA1 and especially BRCA2 mutations are associated with an elevated risk of male breast cancer.

What's the Next Step?

You counsel the patient on obtaining personal genetic testing in light of his family history, in addition to bloodwork evaluation and review of his medication and supplement intake to identify an etiology driving his gynecomastia.

Sequela

The patient submits to testing but fails to follow up with you, although you are able to update him by phone that his genetic testing was positive for a BRCA2 mutation. He returns three years later having lost significant weight due to lifestyle changes but reports that his left breast remains unequally enlarged.

On exam, you notice that there is now a firm immobile mass just below the nipple areola complex. You also palpate an ipsilateral enlarged axillary node.

What's the Working Diagnosis?

At this juncture, a fixed palpable mass is cancer until proven otherwise.

What's the Next Step?

You send the patient for diagnostic bilateral mammography and axillary ultrasound. Based on the results, both the mass and node are biopsied and noted to contain ductal adenocarcinoma, triple receptor negative.

You present his case at a multidisciplinary tumor board. Neoadjuvant chemotherapy followed by total mastectomy is recommended.

Sequela

The patient undergoes neoadjuvant chemotherapy. The tumor seems to decrease in size but the node remains palpable. You consent the patient for modified radical mastectomy, which includes both the total mastectomy and axillary node dissection of levels I and II.

Operative Steps

Total Mastectomy (Fig. 7.1)

1. Incise a large ellipse of skin incorporating the nipple areola complex, leaving only enough for adequate closure.
2. Dissect breast tissue from dermis to the borders of the clavicle, the sternum, the inframammary fold, and the pectoralis muscle.
3. Elevate the breast tissue along with the fascia from the underlying pectoralis.

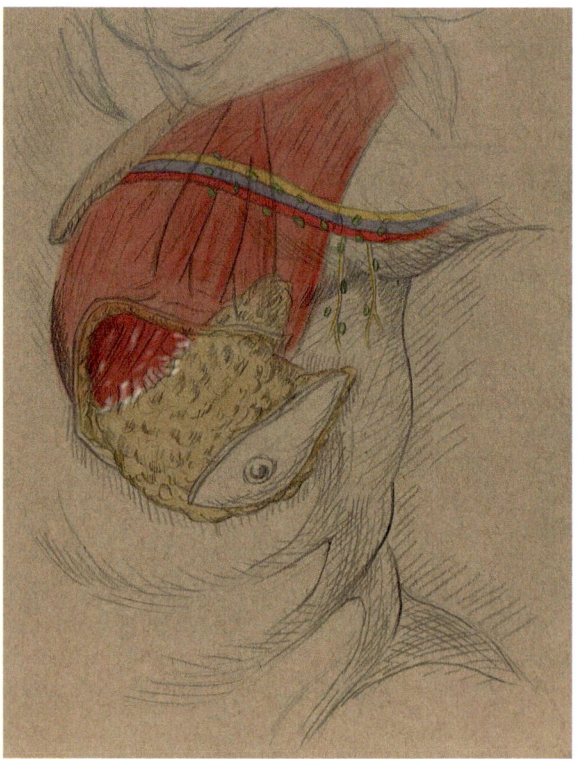

Fig. 7.1 Mastectomy with underlying Rotter's nodes

4. Orient the specimen craniocaudal and mediolateral with sutures.
5. Obtain hemostasis and close the skin flaps over drains.

Axillary Node Dissection for Breast Cancer (Fig. 7.2)

1. Make a transverse incision or carry the mastectomy incision over to the axilla.

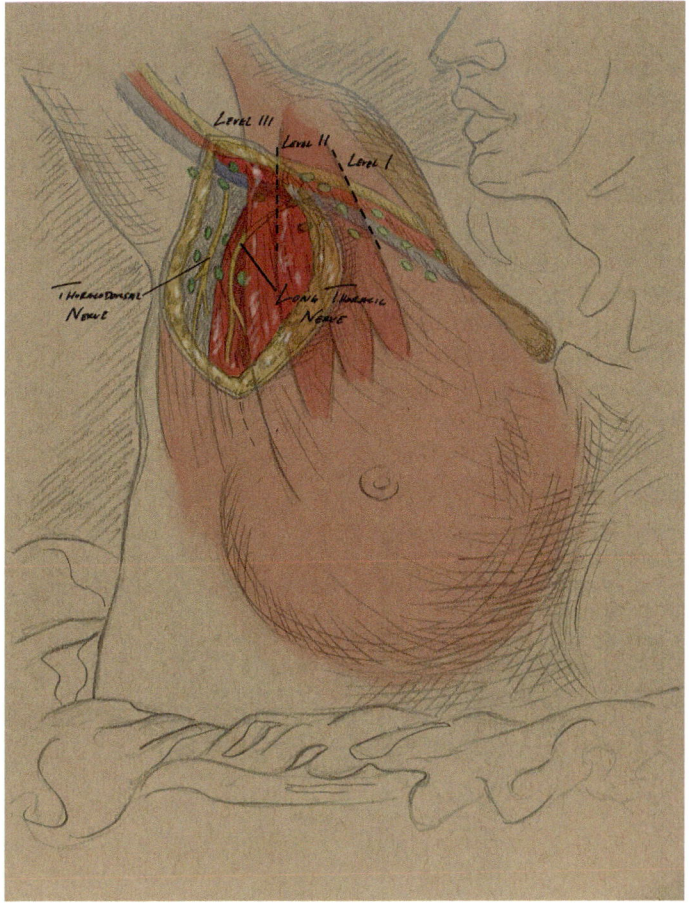

Fig. 7.2 Anatomy of an axillary dissection

2. Free all lymph nodes en bloc from the axillary vein to the latissimus dorsi to the serratus anterior.
3. Include lymph nodes between the pectoralis major and minor muscles (level II).
4. Identify and protect the thoracodorsal nerve and the long thoracic nerve of Bell.
5. Ligate the intercostobrachial nerve if necessary.
6. Obtain hemostasis and close over drains.

The Scenario Changes

Suppose instead of a man, the patient is instead a female who is pregnant in the late second trimester (Table 7.3).

Case Scenario

An 80-year-old woman presents to you for evaluation of nipple discharge. She has noted spontaneous bloody discharge from her right breast, occasionally staining her clothes. She denies pain, palpable lumps or masses, skin changes, or other symptoms. On exam, you are able to express a drop of discharge from a single duct.

Table 7.3 Treatment considerations for a pregnant female with breast cancer

Shield the fetus during mammography
Avoid use of isosulfan blue
Breast conservation is acceptable if the patient can start radiation within 12–16 weeks from surgery
Chemotherapy cannot be given in first trimester
HER2 therapy cannot be given during pregnancy
Hormone therapy cannot be given during pregnancy

What's the Working Diagnosis?

Spontaneous bloody nipple discharge is most likely secondary to a benign papilloma but malignancy must be ruled out. The differential also includes mastitis, duct ectasia, and breast trauma.

What's Your Next Step?

You send the patient for diagnostic mammogram, which only reveals fibrocystic changes. Ultrasound is equally unrevealing. You send the patient for ductography, which reveals a filling defect consistent with a presumptive papilloma. You discuss proceeding with single duct excision.

The Scenario Changes

Suppose you were unable to identify a singular pathologic duct or lesion.

What's the Treatment Plan?

You discuss proceeding with terminal duct excision.

The Scenario Changes

Instead of nipple discharge, your patient presents with a soft new lump in her breast. She feels the lump is a little uncomfortable to touch but denies any skin changes or signs of sepsis. You perform an ultrasound in the office and identify a hypoechoic simple cyst.

What's the Working Diagnosis?

Simple breast cysts are usually benign including oil cyst or fat necrosis, galactocele, or seroma or hematoma. Cysts may also represent abscess or malignancy.

What's the Next Step?

Given that she is symptomatic, you discuss aspirating the fluid. She agrees to proceed. You aspirate the fluid with a needle under ultrasound guidance. The fluid cytology is negative for malignancy.

Additional Reading

1. Giuliano AE, Ballman KV, McCall L, Beitsch PD, Brennan MB, Kelemen PR, Ollila DW, Hansen NM, Whitworth PW, Blumencranz PW, Leitch AM, Saha S, Hunt KK, Morrow M. Effect of axillary dissection vs no axillary dissection on 10-year overall survival among women with invasive breast cancer and sentinel node metastasis: the acosog z0011 (alliance) randomized clinical trial. JAMA. 2017;318(10):918–26. https://doi.org/10.1001/jama.2017.11470. PMID: 28898379; PMCID: PMC5672806.
2. Karamchandani MM, De La Cruz KG, Sokol BL, Chatterjee A, Homsy C. Management of Gynecomastia and Male Benign Diseases. Surg Clin North Am. 2022;102(6):989–1005. https://doi.org/10.1016/j.suc.2022.06.003. PMID: 36335933.
3. National Comprehensive Cancer Network. Breast cancer. In: NCCN clinical practice guidelines in oncology; 2024. https://www.nccn.org/professionals/physician_gls/pdf/breast.pdf. Accessed 30 Dec 2024.
4. Vavolizza RD, Dengel LT. Management of nipple discharge. Surg Clin North Am. 2022;102(6):1077–87. https://doi.org/10.1016/j.suc.2022.06.006. PMID: 36335926.

Vascular

8

Case Scenario

A 73-year-old man presents to the emergency room with acute severe abdominal pain. He has a history of atrial fibrillation and, due to a recent gastrointestinal virus, missed several doses of his rivaroxaban. His abdominal exam is unimpressive but the patient is writhing in pain. His laboratory workup reveals a leukocytosis, a lactic acidosis, and an acute kidney injury.

What's the Working Diagnosis?

In a patient with abdominal "pain out of proportion" to the exam, mesenteric ischemia must be first in consideration. In this particular patient, infectious or inflammatory etiologies are also possible.

You obtain a CT angiogram which confirms not only occlusion to the SMA at its first branch but also demonstrates showered infarcts to the spleen and kidneys.

© The Author(s), under exclusive license to Springer Nature Switzerland AG 2025
S. Hao et al., *General Surgery Boards Case-Based Review*,
https://doi.org/10.1007/978-3-031-85631-0_8

What's the Treatment Plan?

You initiate fluid resuscitation and therapeutic anticoagulation with a heparin infusion. You consent the patient for urgent exploratory laparotomy for SMA embolectomy and possible need for bowel resection.

Operative Steps

SMA Embolectomy

1. Expose the SMA and obtain proximal and distal control (see Chap. 1).
2. Make a transverse arteriotomy and pass a balloon catheter to evacuate distal and proximal clot.
3. Ensure there is adequate backflow and inflow.
4. Repair the arteriotomy after giving a bolus of heparin with running fine monofilament suture.
5. Run the bowel and inspect for perfusion; resect any frankly necrotic segments.
6. Consider temporary closure with second look operation in 24–48 h if there are any questionable portions of bowel.

Sequela

The patient's hemodynamic status improves, the lactic acidosis resolves, but the kidney injury has progressed to renal failure. The nephrologist initiates the patient on hemodialysis via catheter but asks you to evaluate the patient for creation of a natural arteriovenous fistula (AVF). The patient is able to be discharged from the hospital and returns three months later to your office to discuss surgical access options. The patient is right-handed, has never had access procedures or other central lines, and has been tolerating hemodialysis well.

What's Your Next Step?

You clinically assess the arm veins and send the patient for ultrasound examination of the arteries and veins on both arms. The report reveals that both arms have cephalic veins of at least 3 mm from wrist to axilla, however the left radial artery is diminutive and the brachial artery is 2 mm, whereas the right radial artery is 3 mm and the brachial artery is 4 mm.

What's the Treatment Plan?

You discuss with the patient that the left arm vasculature may support a brachiocephalic natural fistula, whereas the right arm could support a radiocephalic natural fistula. You discuss the concepts of going distal to proximal given the expected lifespan of a single dialysis access, as well as the options and expected differences with usage of a prosthetic graft. The patient wishes to proceed with left arm brachiocephalic AVF creation.

Operative Steps

Arteriovenous Fistula Creation of the Arm

1. Position the patient with arm extended under general or regional anesthesia.
2. Make a transverse incision at the antecubital fossa.
3. Isolate and divide the cephalic vein on the radial side of the superficial fossa from its forearm branches, clamping the proximal stump.
4. Incise the antebrachial fascia and identify the brachial artery medial to the biceps tendon.
5. Administer heparin to the patient, clamp the artery distally and proximally, and make an arteriotomy.
6. Spatulate the vein and perform an anastomosis with running fine monofilament nonabsorbable suture.

7. Serially remove clamps and palpate for a thrill.
8. Obtain hemostasis and close in layers.

Sequela

In the recovery room, the patient complains of immediate and severe pain and tingling in the left forearm and hand.

What's the Working Diagnosis?

You are concerned about ischemic monomelic neuropathy. You take the patient back to the operating room for immediate ligation of the access.

The Scenario Changes

The patient experiences an uneventful recovery and returns to the office for follow-up in eight weeks. Their postoperative ultrasound reveals a fistula of 6 mm in diameter, 4 mm under the skin, with flows of 200 cc/min.

What's the Treatment Plan?

You determine that the flow is not yet adequate to support hemodialysis. You opt to reevaluate in four weeks with hopes that the flow may reach closer to 600 cc/min. If the fistula fails to mature, you may have to place a new fistula in another location.

Case Scenario

A 55-year-old woman with heavy tobacco use presents to your office after a recent hospitalization for a stroke. Her primary team obtained a stroke workup while she was hospitalized and identified left-sided carotid artery stenosis. An echocardiogram was negative. She has some residual right arm weakness but is otherwise fully recovered. She is taking aspirin and lisinopril. Her current blood pressure is 140/80 mmHg. The carotid ultrasound indicates 70% stenosis on the left side and < 50% stenosis of the right side.

What's Your Next Step?

You discuss that although asymptomatic stenosis of 70% may not warrant intervention, she has had a stroke and is therefore symptomatic. You counsel her on additional vascular medical management such as starting a statin, quitting smoking, improving her activity level with exercise, consuming a heart-healthy diet, and ensuring optimal blood pressure control. She agrees to optimize her lifestyle and proceed with intervention on her carotid artery stenosis.

Operative Steps

Carotid Artery Exposure (Fig. 8.1)

1. Position the neck extended with head angled away from the operative side.
2. Make an incision parallel to the anterior border of the sternocleidomastoid.
3. Divide the platysma and retract the sternocleidomastoid muscle.
4. Incise the carotid sheath and ligate the facial vein and ansa cervicalis nerve.
5. Identify and protect the vagus nerve and internal jugular vein.

Operative Pearl

Stenting versus endarterectomy is beyond the scope of a general surgeon.

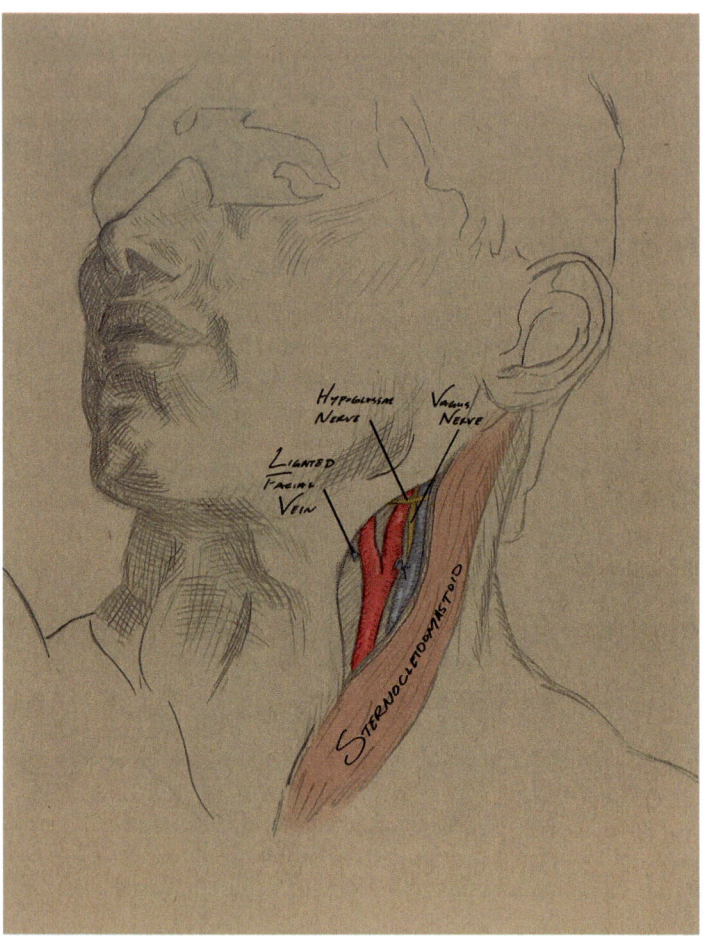

Fig. 8.1 Anatomy of carotid artery exposure

Sequela

You are seeing her in follow-up after carotid artery stenting and she now complains of recent right foot tingling and numbness for several months. She feels that the leg is somewhat cooler than the other leg.

What's the Working Diagnosis?

A patient with one manifestation of vascular disease is likely to have atherosclerosis throughout. Her symptoms may be due to chronic limb ischemia.

What's Your Next Step?

You obtain ankle-brachial indices (ABI) in the office. Her right ABI is 0.6 compared to 0.9 of the left. You also obtain pulse volume recordings which show a dampened waveform distal to the knee. You discuss performing angiography to diagnose and potentially treat a site of occlusion leading to insufficiency.

Sequela

The patient does not wish to proceed. You are called to see the patient several months later in the emergency room with concern for a cold leg. The emergency room physician cannot find a pulse or Doppler signal on the foot. The patient reports significant pain in the leg but is able to weakly flex at the ankle. You confirm lack of foot signals but are able to palpate a femoral pulse. The patient believes she has been having symptoms for over eight hours.

What's the Working Diagnosis?

You are concerned about acute limb ischemia. Although there is no arterial Doppler signal, the limb may be salvageable at this time given there is still motor function (Table 8.1).

Table 8.1   Rutherford classification of acute limb ischemia

Stage	Neuromotor exam	Pulse exam	Next steps
I (no threat)	No deficits	Doppler present	Evaluate if treatment is necessary
IIa (marginal threat)	Sensory deficit	Arterial Doppler loss	Initiate anticoagulation; consider revascularization
IIb (immediate threat)	Sensory and motor deficit	Arterial Doppler loss	Initiate anticoagulation; immediately revascularize
III (irreversible damage)	Sensory loss and paralysis	Arterial and venous Doppler loss	Not salvageable; consider amputation

What's the Treatment Plan?

You initiate the patient on therapeutic anticoagulation and fluid resuscitation and proceed to the operating room for immediate revascularization. Given the prolonged ischemia time, you also consent the patient on the need for fasciotomy.

Operative Steps

Lower Extremity Thrombectomy

1. Prep and drape the lower extremity from hip to foot.
2. Make a vertical incision from lower edge of inguinal ligament at the groin to the apex of the femoral triangle on the medial thigh.
3. Dissect through the fascia to identify the femoral artery and its branches.
4. Obtain vascular control of each branch and the proximal inflow (Fig. 8.2).
5. Administer bolus heparin to the patient and make a transverse arteriotomy on the common femoral artery.

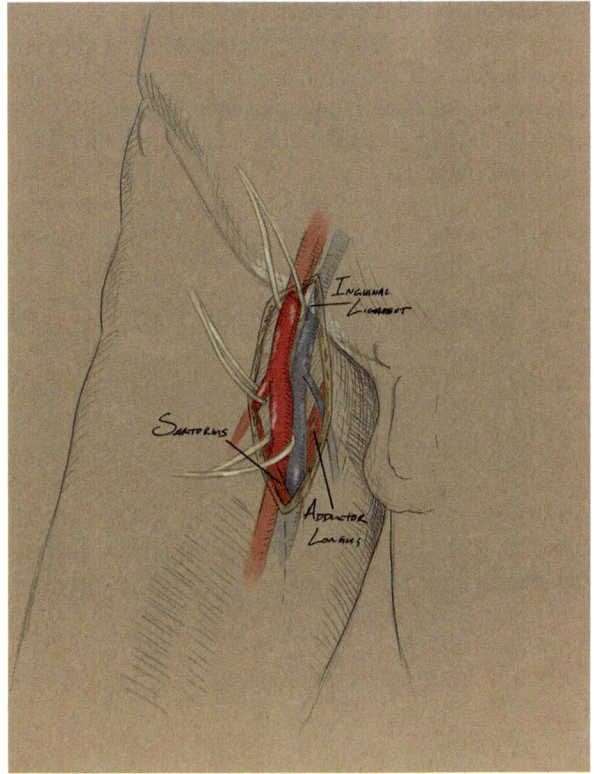

Fig. 8.2 Exposure and control of the femoral arterial vasculature

6. Run a small-caliber balloon catheter down the superficial femoral artery and deep femoral artery until there is adequate backflow and identifiable pedal Doppler signals.
7. Perform femoral endarterectomy if there may be flow-limiting atherosclerotic burden.
8. Close the arteriotomy with running fine monofilament nonabsorbable suture.
9. Close the incision in layers.

Lower Extremity Fasciotomy (Fig. 8.3)

1. Incise the anterolateral leg from between the fibula and tibial
   crest down to the lateral malleolus, approximately 20 cm long.
2. Incise the anterior compartment fascia anterior to the inter-
   muscular septum.

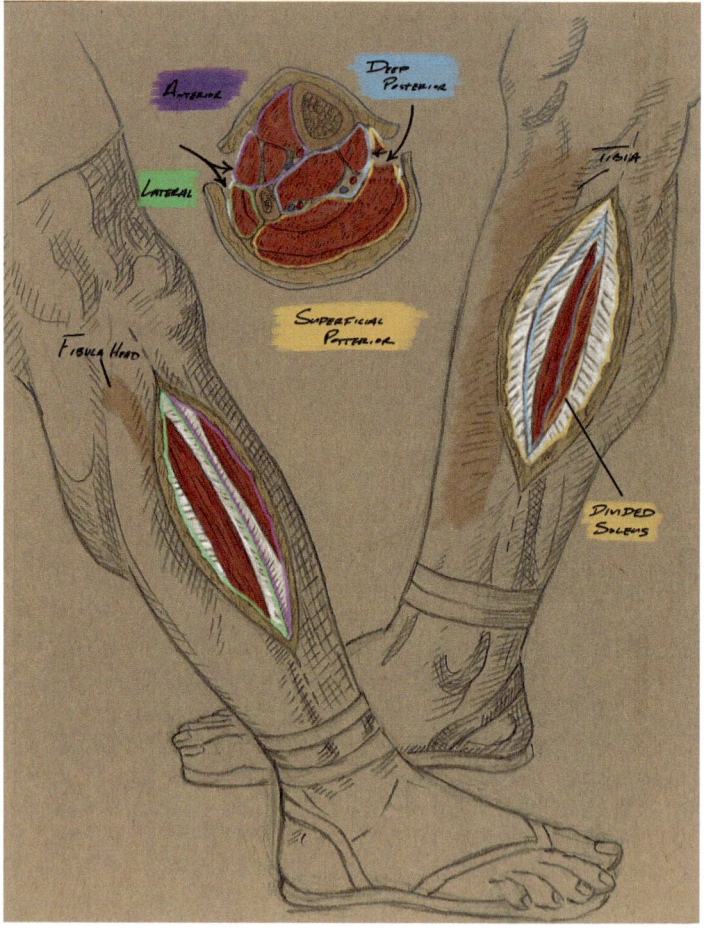

Fig. 8.3 Incisions to open respective compartments of a lower extremity fasciotomy

3. Incise the lateral compartment fascia posterior to the septum, stopping short of the fibular head to protect the common femoral nerve and aiming toward the lateral malleolus to protect the superficial peroneal nerve.
4. Incise the posteromedial leg from the tibial tuberosity to the medial malleolus, approximately 20 cm long.
5. Incise the superficial compartment fascia overlying the gastrocnemius muscle.
6. Incise the soleus fascial bridge and incise the posterior muscle fascia, avoiding the posterior tibial neurovascular bundle between the flexor muscle bodies.
7. Muscle compartments should all visibly bulge.

Sequela

In the ensuing days, despite therapeutic anticoagulation, the pedal signals are lost. The popliteal pulse is maintained. The patient's toes begin to show gangrenous changes. A CT angiogram reveals patent flow until occlusion at the trifurcation.

What's the Treatment Plan?

You discuss lack of distal targets to facilitate a bypass and the need for below knee amputation. The patient reluctantly agrees.

Operative Steps

Below Knee Amputation

1. Prep and drape the lower extremity from hip to foot with an inflated tourniquet on the thigh and a bump under the hip.
2. Make a circumferential incision with fishmouth myocutaneous flaps to cover the eventual stump.
3. Dissect down to the tibia and fibula and elevate the periosteum.

4. Identify, lengthen, and sever each named nerve sharply so to allow retraction.
5. Identify and ligate the associated vascular bundles.
6. Sever the bones with mechanical or automated saw proximal to the skin incision and bevel the sharp edges.
7. Release the tourniquet and obtain hemostasis.
8. Suture the myofascial flaps, followed by the dermis and skin.

Sequela

In the postoperative period, the patient begins to experience waxing and waning episodes of confusion with belligerent behavior.

What's the Working Diagnosis?

Waxing and waning cognitive dysfunction may be hospital delirium, but you obtain workup to rule out organic causes. Bloodwork rules out hypoxia or hypercarbia, electrolyte derangements, nutrient deficiencies, endocrinopathies, and infectious/inflammatory etiologies. Imaging rules out occult stroke, seizure, and cardiomyopathies.

What's the Treatment Plan?

Concluding no organic cause, you then review the medication list and remove or minimize medications that may have cognitive effects, such as narcotics or those on the Beers list. You instruct nursing, ancillary staff, and visiting family to assist with frequent reorientation, daytime activity and nighttime rest, and the provision of familiar items from home, especially medical devices such as glasses or hearing aids.

Case Scenario

A 64-year-old woman presents to the emergency room with painful leg swelling after recent partial colectomy a week ago for an endoscopically unresectable polyp. Her right leg is noticeably edematous and pale. The patient reports the leg is quite painful to move. She is otherwise healthy except for a BMI of 35. She has no personal or family history of blood disorders. She admits to sitting at home in a recliner with little to no activity after her discharge from surgery two days postoperatively. She does have palpable pedal pulses.

What's the Working Diagnosis?

You are primarily concerned about acute deep vein thrombosis with progression to phlegmasia, especially in the setting after major abdominal surgery with increased BMI and potential malignancy of the polyp as well as a sedentary state (Table 8.2).

A duplex ultrasound reveals partially occlusive thrombosis of the common femoral vein. You initiate the patient on therapeutic anticoagulation and admit the patient for close monitoring.

Table 8.2 Differential diagnosis of leg edema

Third-space fluid from heart failure, renal failure, or liver disease
Lymphedema
Deep vein thrombosis
Chronic venous insufficiency

The Scenario Changes

Suppose the patient had a recent hemorrhagic stroke instead of an abdominal surgery.

What's the Treatment Plan?

A recent hemorrhagic stroke would contraindicate initiation of therapeutic anticoagulation. You consult expertise to evaluate the patient for IVC filter placement with or without venous thrombectomy.

Sequela

Suppose the original patient experienced improvement on anticoagulation and was able to be discharged. The thrombotic episode is deemed provoked and the patient is able to discontinue anticoagulation after three months. However, the patient returns to you the following year with persistent leg swelling. A duplex is negative for clot. On exam, there is mild discoloration of the ankle skin and isolated varicosities.

What's the Working Diagnosis?

The venous valves may have become incompetent and are experiencing reflux, otherwise known as insufficiency. You send the patient for repeat ultrasound with instructions to evaluate for reflux. The ultrasound report documents greater than 500 ms of reflux time in the greater saphenous vein.

What's the Treatment Plan?

You counsel the patient on elevating the extremity whenever possible, using graduated compression stockings, and the option for interventions such as vein stripping or vein ablation. The varicosities may be treated with injections or stab phlebectomy but would not resolve the etiology of refluxing veins.

Additional Reading

1. Bowyer MW. Lower extremity fasciotomy: indications and technique. Curr Trauma Rep. 2014;1(1):35–44.
2. Marcantonio ER. Delirium in Hospitalized Older Adults. N Engl J Med. 2017;377(15):1456–66. https://doi.org/10.1056/NEJMcp1605501. PMID: 29020579; PMCID: PMC5706782.
3. Perler AP. Rutherford's vascular surgery and endovascular therapy, 2-volume set. S.L.: Elsevier - Health Science; 2022.
4. Rose DA, Sonaike E, Hughes K. Hemodialysis access. Surg Clin North Am. 2013;93(4):997–1012, x. https://doi.org/10.1016/j.suc.2013.05.002. Epub 2013 Jun 21. PMID: 23885942.

Pediatric

9

Case Scenario

A 3-week-old infant boy presents with bilious vomiting of a few days. The parents report minimal wet diapers and inability to retain any oral intake. The antenatal and perinatal periods were uncomplicated. On exam, the child is lethargic and the fontanelles are depressed. There are no other congenital anomalies identified. Vital signs indicate tachycardia without hypotension. The abdomen is mildly distended but soft and the child fusses when the abdomen is examined. Bloodwork reveals a metabolic alkalosis.

What's the Working Diagnosis?

An infant with bilious vomiting has malrotation until ruled out (Table 9.1).

© The Author(s), under exclusive license to Springer Nature
Switzerland AG 2025
S. Hao et al., *General Surgery Boards Case-Based Review*,
https://doi.org/10.1007/978-3-031-85631-0_9

Table 9.1 Differential diagnosis of emesis in infants

Malrotation with or without volvulus
Hypertrophic pyloric stenosis
Intestinal atresia
Foreign body ingestion
Gastrointestinal infection
Intussusception
Reflux
Meconium ileus
Necrotizing enterocolitis

What's Your Next Step?

You initiate fluid resuscitation and electrolyte correction and order a stat upper GI study. The study reveals contrast passing beyond the pylorus but not crossing midline while in the duodenum. A double bubble is not seen.

What's the Treatment Plan?

Given the diagnostic study, once the child is adequately resuscitated with improvement in the alkalosis, you consent the parents to take the child for exploratory laparotomy with plans for Ladd's procedure.

Operative Steps

Ladd's Procedure

1. Make a transverse incision across the abdomen and eviscerate the bowel.
2. Rotate the bowel in a counterclockwise fashion until the mesentery can be straightened.
3. Release adhesive bands trapping the duodenum to the right abdominal sidewall.
4. Perform an appendectomy.
5. Place the small bowel in the right abdomen and large bowel in the left (Fig. 9.1).

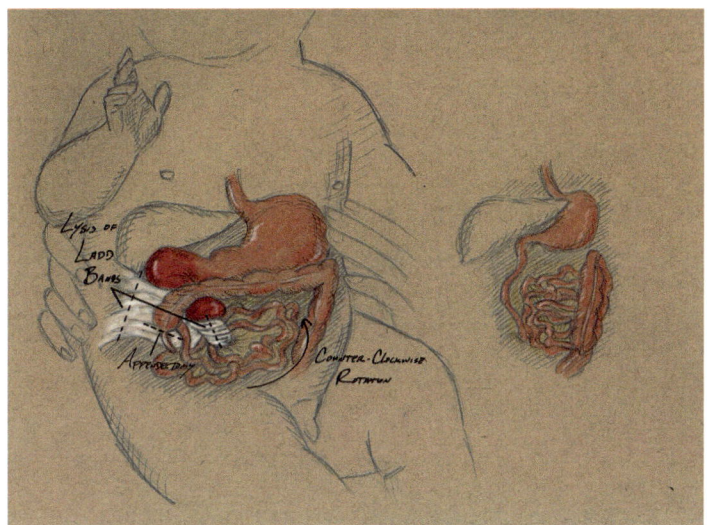

Fig. 9.1 Key steps and final configuration of Ladd's procedure

Operative Pearl

If any of the bowel appears ischemic or questionably so, consider temporizing the abdomen for a second look in 24–48 h prior to proceeding with releasing Ladd's bands.

The Scenario Changes

Suppose the child presents with nonbilious vomiting and the abdominal exam is remarkable for a palpable olive in the midepigastrium. There is a mild alkalosis on bloodwork. Ultrasound demonstrates a long thickened pylorus muscle with obstruction to passage of gastric contents.

What's the Treatment Plan?

This time, you discuss pyloromyotomy with the child's parents and proceed after correction of any fluid and electrolyte deficits.

Operative Steps

Pyloromyotomy (Fig. 9.2)

1. Make an incision in the supraumbilical region.
2. Deliver the stomach and pylorus outside the abdominal cavity.

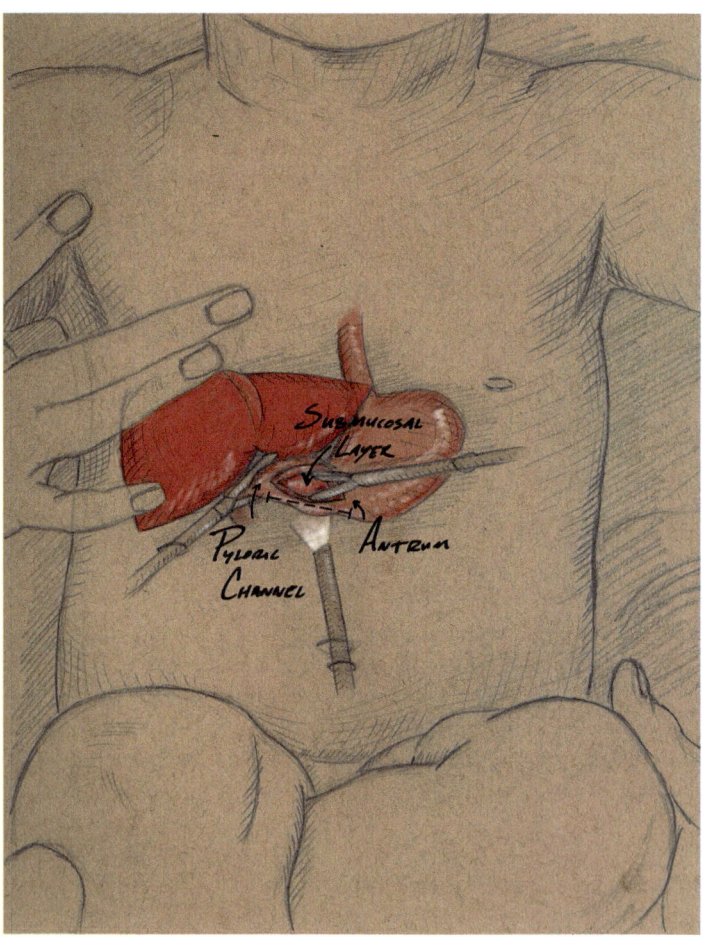

Fig. 9.2 Coronal view of laparoscopic instruments performing pyloromyotomy

3. Incise the pylorus from the antrum to the first portion of the duodenum.
4. Spread the muscle to visualize mucosal bulging.
5. Confirm no mucosal violation.
6. After confirming no other intra-abdominal pathology, close the abdomen.

Operative Pearl

If the mucosa is violated, it is acceptable to either simply repair the mucosa with or without an omental patch or completely repair the mucosal and muscle defect and perform the myotomy on the other side. An upper gastrointestinal series can be obtained prior to feeding postoperatively.

Sequela

Postoperatively, you admit the patient for monitoring for postoperative apnea or bradycardia, with a plan to administer clear liquids first and then progress to full feeds with proven tolerance.

The child continues to have nonbilious vomiting five days after surgery.

What's the Working Diagnosis?

An incomplete pyloromyotomy is possible although it may be too soon to tell. You opt to continue supportive care with plans for repeat pyloromyotomy if emesis persists beyond a week.

Case Scenario

A 15-month-old girl presents to the emergency room with bloody stools. This was preceded by colicky abdominal pain without particular localization. Bloodwork is largely unremarkable. The parents describe the stools as red jelly-like. An abdominal ultrasound identifies a target sign in the right lower quadrant.

What's the Working Diagnosis?

The clinical picture indicates intussusception. You discuss proceeding with an enema reduction by the radiologist, followed by a period of observation. The parents consent to proceed. The enema reduction is successful, but hours later, the patient again develops the same colicky pain.

What's the Treatment Plan?

Given the recurrent symptoms, the intussusception likely recurred. The radiologist agrees to try a second attempt at enema reduction. The second attempt is unsuccessful. You discuss proceeding with surgical reduction.

Operative Steps

Surgical Reduction of Pediatric Intussusception

1. Access the abdominal cavity via transverse incision in the right lower quadrant or laparoscopic port sites akin to an appendectomy procedure.
2. Manually push the intussusceptum retrograde out of the intussuscipiens.
3. Inspect the bowel for perforation or necrosis.
4. Carefully examine the bowel for a lead point.
5. Consider appendectomy if a right lower quadrant incision was used.

Intraoperatively, you identify a wide-based Meckel's diverticulum while searching for a lead point.

What's the Treatment Plan?

Although Meckel's may be an innocent bystander, it can also be a lead point for intussusception or a source for heterotopic mucosa leading to lower GI bleeding in children. You speak with the parents by phone to discuss the risks and benefits of proceeding with Meckel's diverticulectomy. The parents wish to have it removed.

> **Operative Pearl**
>
> There is no agreed-upon method of Meckel's diverticulectomy. It is possible to resect with stapler or with sharp transection followed by transverse suture closure of the ileum. It is also valid to resect the portion of the ileum containing Meckel's and perform primary anastomosis if doing otherwise may leave behind ulcerated mucosa or a narrowed lumen.

Case Scenario

A 6-month-old baby boy born prematurely is referred to your office. The parents have noticed both persistence of an umbilical hernia present at birth and bilateral groin swelling when the baby cries. On exam, you confirm all three hernia defects but also note a firm palpable mass in the left hemiabdomen.

What's the Working Diagnosis?

A solid abdominal mass in the infant is concerning for malignancy (Table 9.2).

Table 9.2 Differential diagnosis of a solid abdominal mass in a pediatric patient

Lymphoma
Neuroblastoma
Wilms' tumor (nephroblastoma)
Hepatoblastoma
Germ cell tumor
Sarcoma

A CT scan is concerning for a Wilms' tumor. Bloodwork is negative for cytopenias, catecholamine elevation, germ cell tumor markers, or electrolyte derangements. Physical exam and additional imaging are negative for congenital anomalies. You refer the patient to appropriate specialists for further care.

The Scenario Changes

The child does not have an abdominal mass but still has all three hernias.

What's the Treatment Plan?

You discuss proceeding with elective bilateral inguinal hernia repair. Done laparoscopically, you may also repair the umbilical hernia at the same time.

Operative Steps

Pediatric Inguinal Hernia Repair

1. Make a transverse incision over the groin lateral to the pubic tubercle.
2. Dissect down to the external ring.
3. Incise the external oblique aponeurosis from the external ring up if necessary, taking care not to injure the nearby genitofemoral nerve.
4. Free the hernia sac from the cord structures and reduce any hernia contents.
5. Ligate the sac at the internal ring and then resect the sac.
6. Repair the aponeurosis and reconstruct the external ring.
7. Close the wound in layers and confirm scrotal location of the ipsilateral testicle.

The Scenario Changes

This time, the child only has an umbilical hernia which is asymptomatic.

What's the Treatment Plan?

You counsel the parents on signs and symptoms of incarceration but defer repair until the child is five years old, since pediatric umbilical hernias may spontaneously close up to that point.

Additional Reading

1. Abdulhai S, Glenn IC, Ponsky TA. Inguinal hernia. Clin Perinatol. 2017;44(4):865–77. https://doi.org/10.1016/j.clp.2017.08.005. Epub 2017 Sep 20. PMID: 29127966.
2. Charles T, Penninga L, Reurings JC, Berry MC. Intussusception in children: a clinical review. Acta Chir Belg. 2015;115(5):327–33. https://doi.org/10.1080/00015458.2015.11681124. PMID: 26559998.
3. Hansen CC, Søreide K. Systematic review of epidemiology, presentation, and management of Meckel's diverticulum in the twenty-first century. Medicine (Baltimore). 2018;97(35):e12154. https://doi.org/10.1097/MD.0000000000012154. PMID: 30170459; PMCID: PMC6392637.
4. Millar AJ, Rode H, Cywes S. Malrotation and volvulus in infancy and childhood. Semin Pediatr Surg. 2003;12(4):229–36. https://doi.org/10.1053/j.sempedsurg.2003.08.003. PMID: 14655161.
5. Rentea RM, Peter SDS, Snyder CL. Pediatric appendicitis: state of the art review. Pediatr Surg Int. 2017;33(3):269–83. https://doi.org/10.1007/s00383-016-3990-2. Epub 2016 Oct 14. PMID: 27743024.
6. Zaghal A, El-Majzoub N, Jaafar R, Aoun B, Jradi N. Brief overview and updates on infantile hypertrophic pyloric stenosis: focus on perioperative management. Pediatr Ann. 2021;50(3):e136–41. https://doi.org/10.3928/19382359-20210215-01. Epub 2021 Mar 1. PMID: 34038653.

Endocrine

10

Case Scenario

You are called to see a 39-year-old man admitted to the medical intensive care unit with acute pancreatitis. Alcohol consumption has been deemed the etiology. He has been fluid resuscitated but due to ongoing clinical symptoms and worsening leukocytosis, a repeat CT scan was obtained which showed areas of necrosis without gas.

What's the Working Diagnosis?

Without gas, you presume there is sterile pancreatic necrosis. You discuss proceeding with a step-up approach (Table 10.1).

© The Author(s), under exclusive license to Springer Nature Switzerland AG 2025
S. Hao et al., *General Surgery Boards Case-Based Review*, https://doi.org/10.1007/978-3-031-85631-0_10

Table 10.1 Step-up approach for necrotizing pancreatitis

Percutaneous or endoscopic transgastric drainage
Video-assisted retroperitoneal debridement or endoscopic necrosectomy
Open necrosectomy

Sequela

The patient improves after percutaneous drainage and the drain is removed. He returns to your office six weeks later with residual persistent discomfort and early satiety. A repeat CT scan reveals a walled-off persistent 5 cm fluid collection in the tail of the pancreas adjacent to the stomach wall.

What's the Working Diagnosis?

Although cystic lesions in the pancreas may represent malignancy such as cystic neoplasms, a pseudocyst is most likely in the immediate setting after an episode of acute pancreatitis.

What's the Treatment Plan?

A symptomatic walled-off pseudocyst is amenable to intervention once it has matured at 4–6 weeks. This can be done with percutaneous drainage or endoscopic or surgical cystgastrostomy if the stomach is in proximity.

The Scenario Changes

The patient instead presents to you years later with watery secretory diarrhea associated with weight loss. His primary physician obtained a CT scan demonstrating a 3.5 cm mass in the pancreatic tail. Bloodwork reveals low potassium and elevated calcium.

Table 10.2 Differential diagnosis of a pancreatic mass

Pancreatic adenocarcinoma
Cystic neoplasms including mucinous cystic neoplasms, serous
cystadenoma, intraductal papillary mucinous neoplasms, and solid
pseudopapillary neoplasms
Neuroendocrine tumors including glucagonoma, insulinoma, VIPoma,
gastrinoma
Metastatic lesion

What's the Working Diagnosis?

Based on the clinical symptoms and lab values, you are concerned for a functional endocrine tumor in the pancreas, possibly a VIPoma (Table 10.2).

What's Your Next Step?

You obtain a panel of bloodwork including VIP levels and an octreotide scan given your suspicion. Your workup is consistent with VIPoma. You obtain a full family history to rule out genetic syndromes. You initiate the patient on octreotide and discuss distal pancreatectomy with splenectomy pending response to octreotide. The patient inquires about a less invasive option. You counsel the patient that enucleation is acceptable for smaller tumors at a distance from the pancreatic duct and for tumors that have low malignant potential. The size of his tumor precludes him from enucleation.

Operative Steps

Distal Pancreatectomy and Splenectomy (Fig. 10.1)

1. Mobilize the splenic flexure and enter the lesser sac to visualize the pancreatic tail.
2. Divide the splenic hilum and free the spleen from its attachments.

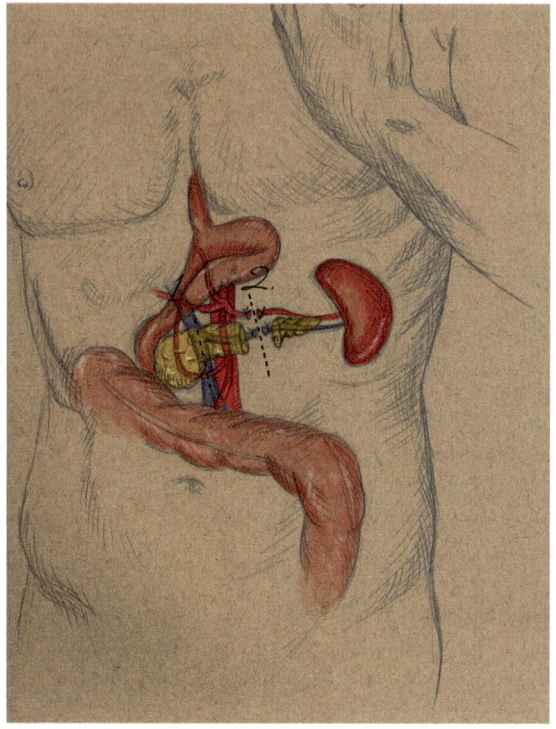

Fig. 10.1 Central and distal pancreatectomy as defined by the SMA

3. Mobilize the inferior border of the pancreas.
4. Staple across the pancreatic body proximal to the tumor.
5. Elevate the specimen from the retroperitoneum.
6. Obtain hemostasis and leave a drain.

Operative Pearl

The literature would suggest that outcomes are not different for pancreatic neuroendocrine tumors treated with spleen-preserving distal pancreatectomy. However, including the spleen is necessary for an oncologic resection if there is any concern for malignant potential (Fig. 10.2).

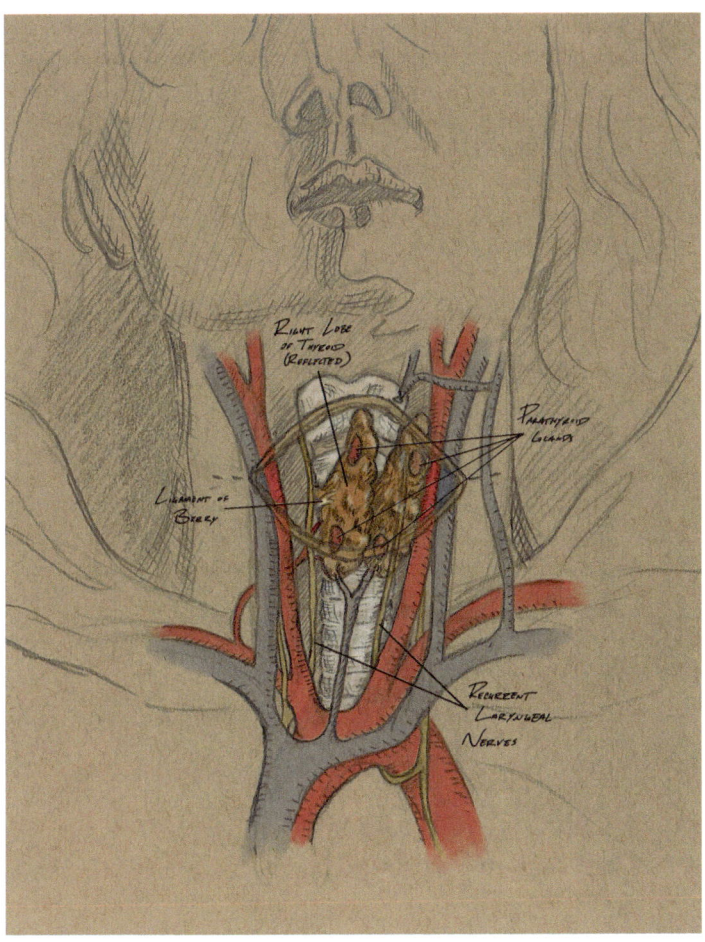

Fig. 10.2 Medial view of the right lobe of the thyroid with its parathyroids

Case Scenario

A 51-year-old woman presents in referral to your office for incidentally noted blood calcium level of 11.5 mg/dL. She has had a kidney stone recently managed conservatively. She has a negative family history. She does not take any medications or supplements.

What's Your Next Step?

You obtain a parathyroid hormone (PTH) level which is elevated.

What's the Working Diagnosis?

This patient has hypercalcemia from hyperparathyroidism, which is likely from an adenoma in the setting of normal renal function. Due to her history of stones, she meets criteria for surgery (Table 10.3). You discuss removal of the offending parathyroid.

Table 10.3 Indications for parathyroidectomy for primary hypercalcemia

Patient age < 50
Serum calcium > 1 mg/dL over the upper limit of normal
Urinary calcium loss > 400 mg/day
Kidney stones
Osteopenia with a Z score less than 2
Renal disease
Neuromuscular symptoms from hypercalcemia

What's the Treatment Plan?

You obtain a sestamibi scan for operative planning. The scan highlights a singular adenoma on the right.

Operative Steps

Parathyroidectomy

1. With the patient supine, neck extended, and set up for nerve monitoring, make a collar incision 1–2 fingerbreadths above the sternal notch.
2. Divide and elevate platysmal flaps.
3. Incise the median raphe and retract the strap muscles.
4. Obtain a baseline PTH blood level prior to manipulating the glands.
5. Reflect the thyroid lobe medially, dividing the middle thyroid vein (Table 10.2).
6. Identify both superior and inferior parathyroids and resect if abnormal in appearance.
7. Obtain a post-resection PTH blood level after 15 min.
8. Obtain hemostasis and close in layers.

Operative Pearl

If the PTH does not fall appropriately (more than 50% or into normal range) or none of the parathyroids appear abnormal, it is necessary to perform four-gland exploration.

The Scenario Changes

While working up the patient, the PTH level is in fact suppressed. You check a parathyroid hormone-related protein (PTHRP) level which is elevated.

What's the Working Diagnosis?

You are concerned for pseudohyperparathyroidism due to a paraneoplastic process. You obtain cross-sectional imaging to identify a primary malignancy. A left lung lesion in the distal tip of the upper lobe is found associated with a pleural effusion.

You consult the oncology team, who requests sampling of the effusion for cytology, as the interventional radiologists are currently absent.

Operative Steps

Thoracentesis

1. Position the patient upright and leaning forward.
2. Confirm a window of fluid under ultrasound guidance.
3. Inject local anesthetic at the planned site of insertion, distal to the scapular tip.
4. Insert the needle while withdrawing until fluid is aspirated.
5. If placing a catheter, perform this with Seldinger technique over wire.
6. Cover with occlusive dressing and obtain a post-procedure plain film.

The cytology is uninformative and the interventional radiologists remain unavailable. To obtain a diagnosis, the oncology team requests a biopsy.

Operative Steps

Video-Assisted Thoracoscopy and Wedge Resection

1. Position the patient in lateral decubitus with flexion.
2. With the patient on single lung ventilation, place triangulated ports in the midaxillary line in the seventh intercostal space,

anterior to the scapular tip, and in the fourth intercostal space in the anterior axillary line (Fig. 10.3).

3. Grasp the intended specimen and perform a staple wedge resection.

4. Place apical and basilar chest tubes and reinflate the lung under direct visualization.

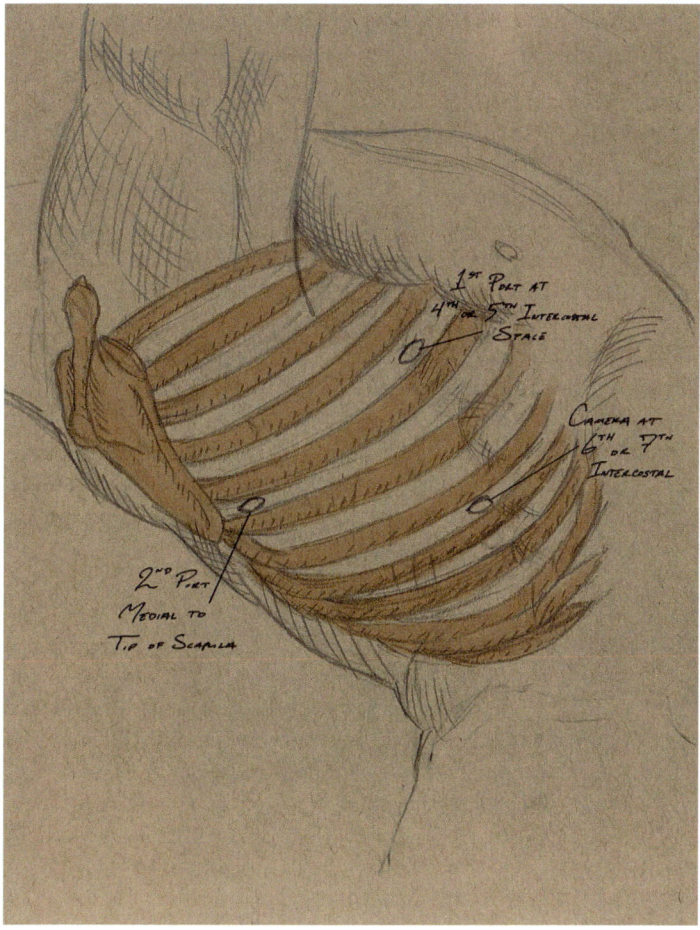

Fig. 10.3 Port placement for thoracoscopy

5. Close over the chest tubes with occlusive dressing and obtain post-procedural plain films.

> **Operative Pearl**
>
> Although there is no agreement on the utility of plain films after removing chest tubes, have a defined practice pattern on criteria to remove a chest tube and criteria to monitor or image for reaccumulated pneumothorax after chest tube removal.

Sequela

In the immediate postoperative period, the nurse calls you to see the patient for an arrhythmia. An EKG reveals irregularly irregular atrial beats with rapid ventricular rate. The systolic blood pressure is 105 mmHg.

What's the Working Diagnosis?

You are concerned about post-pulmonary resection atrial fibrillation. Given that the patient is not unstable, you start with chemical cardioversion with amiodarone bolus followed by infusion. Beta-blockade may also be necessary.

The Scenario Changes

During initial evaluation, the patient reports hearing that several family members underwent thyroid surgery and adrenal resection for cancer, although she herself is unaware of any genetic testing and unaware of the final diagnoses.

What's the Working Diagnosis?

You are concerned that the patient may have a genetic disorder such as the multiple endocrine neoplasia syndromes. The patient consents to genetic testing. In the meantime, you obtain a neck ultrasound which does show a 9 mm thyroid mass but no abnormal adenopathy. Fine needle aspiration cytology reports Bethesda V, suspicious for medullary cancer. You also send off catecholamine serum levels, which are elevated, and tumor markers including calcitonin and CEA, both of which are also elevated.

What's Your Next Step?

You obtain 24-h urine catecholamine levels to confirm a true elevation and then obtain CT imaging to identify an adrenal lesion. There is a 4 cm enhancing lesion with delayed washout in the right adrenal gland.

What's the Treatment Plan?

With this constellation of findings, you plan on sequentially treating the patient. You address the pheochromocytoma first by initiating alpha- followed by beta-blockade, with plans to perform adrenalectomy once adequate hemodynamic control has been achieved. Following this, you plan on a total thyroidectomy with 3.5 gland parathyroidectomy with autotransplantation.

Operative Steps

Right Adrenalectomy

1. Access the abdominal cavity with a transverse subcostal incision.
2. Mobilize the hepatic flexure of the colon and the liver itself after dividing ligamentous attachments.
3. Divide Gerota's fascia to identify the adrenal gland.
4. Clip and divide the adrenal vein from the IVC with appropriate communication to the anesthesia team.
5. Mobilize and divide the investing tissue along with its feeding arterial supply with an energy device.
6. Obtain hemostasis and close the incision in layers.

> **Operative Pearl**
>
> A tumor smaller than 6 cm can be approached laparoscopically, either through the flank or through the peritoneal cavity.

Sequela

The patient has persistent postoperative hypotension without signs of hemorrhage, in addition to lethargy and generalized weakness. An infectious workup is equally unrevealing.

What's the Working Diagnosis?

Although more common after resection of cortisol-secreting tumors or in patients on glucocorticoid supplementation, adrenal insufficiency remains a possibility after adrenalectomy.

What's Your Next Step?

You order a cosyntropin stimulation test, with cortisol levels checked before and 30 min after administration of 250 mcg of cosyntropin. If the baseline is low and does not appropriately rise after stimulation, you initiate the patient on 100 mg IV hydrocortisone every eight hours.

Sequela

The patient recovers from this operation and is ready to proceed with thyroid surgery.

Operative Steps

Total Thyroidectomy

1. With the patient supine, neck extended, and set up for nerve monitoring, make a collar incision 1–2 fingerbreadths above the sternal notch.
2. Divide and elevate platysmal flaps.
3. Incise the median raphe and retract the strap muscles.
4. Mobilize the thyroid lobes sequentially, ligating the middle thyroid vein.
5. Divide the thyroid ligamentous attachments superiorly and inferiorly and elevate from the pretracheal fascia.
6. Identify and protect the recurrent laryngeal nerve throughout the dissection.
7. Dice the most normal-appearing parathyroid gland, no more than 50 g of tissue, and place in a pocket of vascularized muscle such as the sternocleidomastoid.
8. Close the incision in layers over a drain.

Sequela

You initiate the patient postoperatively on thyroid hormone replacement therapy in addition to calcium replacement therapy. You surveil the patient with annual tumor markers and catecholamines and monitor thyroid hormone, PTH, and calcium levels.

Case Scenario

A 22-year-old woman presents with acute abdominal pain in the right lower quadrant. She believes she has missed her period. She has had a prior appendectomy. Her beta-human chorionic gonadotropin (beta-hCG) levels are elevated. She is mildly tachycardic but normotensive.

What's the Working Diagnosis?

The elevated hormone levels suggest active pregnancy, which in the setting of pain may be due to miscarriage or ectopic site of implantation. Other gynecologic as well as gastrointestinal causes of adnexal pain are also possibilities, including appendicitis, diverticulitis, ovarian cyst rupture, ovarian torsion, and pelvic inflammatory disease.

What's Your Next Step?

You obtain a transvaginal ultrasound which confirms no intrauterine pregnancy and identifies a fetal heartbeat outside the uterine cavity.

What's the Treatment Plan?

In an otherwise stable and uncomplicated setting, you discuss termination of the ectopic pregnancy with methotrexate.

The Scenario Changes

The same patient upon return from the transvaginal ultrasound decompensates with worsening tachycardia and hypotension, with an abdominal exam concerning for peritonitis. A rapid bedside ultrasound indicates free abdominal fluid.

What's the Working Diagnosis?

The concern is now for ruptured ectopic pregnancy. You quickly discuss the need for surgical intervention with the patient, indicating the potential for possible removal of the fallopian tube.

Operative Steps

Laparoscopic Salpingostomy or Salpingectomy

1. Access and insufflate the abdomen and place ports in the umbilicus and suprapubic region.
2. Identify the site of ectopic pregnancy and incise the fallopian tube longitudinally on the anti-mesenteric surface.
3. Extract the products of conception and consider suturing close the incision.
4. If unable to safely preserve the fallopian tube, staple and resect the fallopian tube from the ectopic site to the fimbria.

Additional Reading

1. National Comprehensive Cancer Network. Thyroid carcinoma. In: NCCN clinical practice guidelines in oncology; 2024. https://www.nccn.org/professionals/physician_gls/pdf/thyroid.pdf. Accessed 30 Dec 2024.
2. Po L, Thomas J, Mills K, Zakhari A, Tulandi T, Shuman M, Page A. Guideline No. 414: management of pregnancy of unknown location and tubal and Nontubal ectopic pregnancies. J Obstet Gynaecol Can. 2021;43(5):614–630.e1. https://doi.org/10.1016/j.jogc.2021.01.002. Epub 2021 Jan 13. PMID: 33453378.
3. Rivers EP, Gaspari M, Saad GA, Mlynarek M, Fath J, Horst HM, Wortsman J. Adrenal insufficiency in high-risk surgical ICU patients. Chest. 2001;119(3):889–96. https://doi.org/10.1378/chest.119.3.889. PMID: 11243973.
4. Uludağ M, Aygün N, İşgör A. Surgical Indications and Techniques for Adrenalectomy. Sisli Etfal Hastan Tip Bul. 2020;54(1):8–22. https://doi.org/10.14744/SEMB.2019.05578. PMID: 32377128; PMCID: PMC7192258.
5. van Santvoort HC, Besselink MG, Bakker OJ, Hofker HS, Boermeester MA, Dejong CH, van Goor H, Schaapherder AF, van Eijck CH, Bollen TL, van Ramshorst B, Nieuwenhuijs VB, Timmer R, Laméris JS, Kruyt PM, Manusama ER, van der Harst E, van der Schelling GP, Karsten T, Hesselink EJ, van Laarhoven CJ, Rosman C, Bosscha K, de Wit RJ, Houdijk AP, van Leeuwen MS, Buskens E, Gooszen HG, Dutch Pancreatitis Study Group. A step-up approach or open necrosectomy for necrotizing pancreatitis. N Engl J Med. 2010;362(16):1491–502. https://doi.org/10.1056/NEJMoa0908821. PMID: 20410514.

6. Wilhelm SM, Wang TS, Ruan DT, Lee JA, Asa SL, Duh QY, Doherty GM, Herrera MF, Pasieka JL, Perrier ND, Silverberg SJ, Solórzano CC, Sturgeon C, Tublin ME, Udelsman R, Carty SE. The American Association of Endocrine Surgeons Guidelines for Definitive Management of Primary Hyperparathyroidism. JAMA Surg. 2016;151(10):959–68. https://doi.org/10.1001/jamasurg.2016.2310. PMID: 27532368.
7. Ziarnik E, Grogan EL. Postlobectomy Early Complications. Thorac Surg Clin. 2015;25(3):355–64. https://doi.org/10.1016/j.thorsurg.2015.04.003. Epub 2015 Jun 12. PMID: 26210931; PMCID: PMC4606870

Index